# SpringerBriefs in Psychology

SpringerBriefs present concise summaries of cutting-edge research and practical applications across a wide spectrum of fields. Featuring compact volumes of 55 to 125 pages, the series covers a range of content from professional to academic. Typical topics might include:

- A timely report of state-of-the-art analytical techniques
- A bridge between new research results as published in journal articles and a contextual literature review
- A snapshot of a hot or emerging topic
- An in-depth case study or clinical example
- A presentation of core concepts that readers must understand to make independent contributions

SpringerBriefs in Psychology showcase emerging theory, empirical research, and practical application in a wide variety of topics in psychology and related fields. Briefs are characterized by fast, global electronic dissemination, standard publishing contracts, standardized manuscript preparation and formatting guidelines, and expedited production schedules.

Kamilla Varsha Rawatlal

# Clinical Supervision in South Africa

Improving practice with limited resources

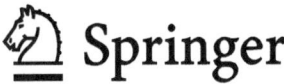 Springer

Kamilla Varsha Rawatlal
University of Pretoria
Pretoria East, South Africa

ISSN 2192-8363          ISSN 2192-8371   (electronic)
SpringerBriefs in Psychology
ISBN 978-3-031-41928-7          ISBN 978-3-031-41929-4   (eBook)
https://doi.org/10.1007/978-3-031-41929-4

This Springer imprint is published by the registered company Springer Nature Switzerland AG
The registered company address is: Gewerbestrasse 11, 6330 Cham, Switzerland

Paper in this product is recyclable.

*This book is dedicated to trainee practitioners and clinical supervisors who navigate the complexities and challenges of mental health provision in resource constrained contexts.*

# Preface

The book represents my account of transition from practitioner, clinical supervisor to academia against the backdrop of serving at public health and educational institutions. In documenting my accounts, though integrating a systematic lens, it is hoped that trainees and established practitioners as well as clinical supervisors in the field of mental health care will strengthen their knowledge base, competence and confidence in navigating the sometimes challenging and unpredictable terrain of practice in public settings. The aim and the scope of this publication is to provide the reader (trainee Health Professionals and practitioners) with a resource and a self-directed supervisory guide, which they can engage in reflection at the different systemic levels to inform navigating complex and resource constrained contexts where there are sometimes no clinical supervisors readily available. By engaging the reader in such a structured and systematic process of clinical supervision, through the ecological model, it is envisaged that practitioners will develop skills and competencies to increase their resilience in resource-constrained contexts. This, in turn, will facilitate better treatment and management plans for their clients and patients.

The focus on a systematic approach allows the book to be pragmatic in seeking solutions to contemporary challenges and realities in practice settings. It has been the experience that such realities speak largely to practitioners' resilience and hence the need turns the lens inward and addresses practitioner's innate humanness (level of the core), self-reflection and wellbeing before addressing competence to serve as behavioural scientist practitioners. Implicit in the systematic approach advocated is a framework that seeks addressing competence at multiple levels. It is with this in mind that I have attempted to provide a structured, guided approach to support practitioners' process and integrate both the personal and professional in the development of their identity as professionals.

Included in this publication is a focus on practitioners and clinical supervisors' self-care and wellbeing, which has been regarded as a neglected area in training. I pay gratitude to Professor Tharina Guse (Counselling Psychologist, Head of Department of Psychology, Department of Psychology, University of Pretoria), whose work sheds much light on this area for trainee's and trainee practitioners. I also pay gratitude to Professor Inge Petersen (Counselling Psychologist, Director of the Centre for Rural Health, College of Health Sciences, University of KwaZulu-Natal) who influenced my conceptualisation of the application and relevance of ecological systemic approaches to mental health intervention in scarce resource contexts.

As I conclude writing this publication in the month of April, which has been regarded as an extraordinary month of giving as it marks the auspicious period of Ramadan, Lent, Easter, Ram Navami and Passover, it is hoped that readers of all faiths derive reflection on their practice from this book and be reminded of our common good and humanity in continuing to serve all patients and clients with the utmost integrity, dignity and respect!

Pretoria East, South Africa                                             Kamilla Varsha Rawatlal

# Contents

# List of Figures

# List of Tables

# Chapter 1
# Introduction and Background to Institutions of Practice

## 1.1 Introduction

In this book, the author advocates for integrating an ecological, systemic framework to support practitioners (level one Masters' students, interns and Health Professionals) navigate twenty-first-century challenges and opportunities in the provision of mental health care services at various institutions in developing countries such as South Africa. With an increased uptake of mental health care services in recent times, post the COVID-19 pandemic; the advent of telepsychology; the need to make mental health care services more accessible; the need to integrate indigenous knowledge and skills (IKS) in diverse contexts, health care professionals have had to reconcile working within institutional structures that place increased challenges and pressures. Psychologists and Health Professionals employed in various resource-constrained settings such as governmental institutions such as the health care sector and higher education institutions have been subject to multiple competing demands that increase the risk of compassion fatigue and burnout.

Research has demonstrated that burnout emerges from multiple institutional, professional and personal factors, including health professional's beliefs and coping abilities. The focus of this book is on building the capacity of mental health professionals to navigate both opportunities and challenges that these contexts present. Through focusing on the different ecological levels that influence professional's identity, namely the intrapersonal (individual level attributes and competencies), the interpersonal (professional identity development in relation to reflecting on self, others, and the influence of models of psychotherapy) and the institutional (professionals ability to navigate the external), the author provides a framework for integrating the multiple levels that influence health professional's professional identity development with a view to support navigating and adjusting to twenty-first-century realities,

© The Author(s), under exclusive license to Springer Nature Switzerland AG 2023
K. V. Rawatlal, *Clinical Supervision in South Africa*, SpringerBriefs in Psychology,
https://doi.org/10.1007/978-3-031-41929-4_1

The work of Falender and Shafranske (2017) has provided great impetus for highlighting that in the field competency-based clinical supervision, competency is constantly evolving and developing, further clinicians or supervisors never achieve absolute competence. The reality, they indicate, is that our own competence is fleeting because the field continuously advances knowledge and professional practices (Falender & Shafranske, 2017). It is with this in mind that we invite the reader (both experienced and at the level of trainee) to use this publication to better support practice and intervention in the twenty-first century for clients and patients from all walks of life that it was intended for.

To provide a summary of the chapters, in *Chap. 1,* the author begins with integrating an ecological systemic framework to support practitioners navigate twenty-first-century challenges through contextualising different institutions of practice of health professionals. The author locates different 'zones' of practice as Zone A – Institutions of Higher Learning and Zone B – The Health Care System.

In *Chap. 2, The Evolution of Supervisory Models,* I present a brief overview of the defining features and evolution of traditional models of clinical supervision. Psychoanalytic, Cognitive Behavioural, Person Centred, Narrative and Integrated approaches are explored with a view to also understand application issues in contemporary practice. The need to integrate indigenous knowledge and skills in culturally complex and diverse countries such as South Africa, to serve the different ethnic groups, i.e. African, Indian, White, and Afrikaans speaking to provide holistic treatment and management plans is also explored.

In *Chap. 3, Towards a Systemic and Relational Ecological Framework to Clinical Supervision,* I present a conceptualisation of integrating an ecological framework to clinical supervision. This chapter begins with laying the theoretical foundation of the ecological, systemic framework and the different levels that will inform a systemic, methodical and systematic approach to supporting trainee health professionals/health professionals navigating practice realities. In *Chap. 4, Level One: The Core: Informing Supervisee's Internal Lens of Reference,* the author discusses informing the first level or the core in practitioner development. The individual level characteristics (personality strengths and weaknesses, worldview, attitude, motivation, identity as a professional) of supervisees are explored. *Chapter 5, Supervisee's Interpersonal Frame of Reference,* the author discusses the supervisee's interpersonal frame of reference and draws attention to the supervisee interacting through the process of self-awareness, self-reflection, reflexivity with the supervisor and the various therapeutic approaches and interventions. Incorporating 'resilience-based approaches' and reflective inventories to strengthen supervisees self-awareness is also drawn.

In *Chap. 6, Navigating the External (Institutional)*, I discuss supporting trainee professionals in navigating the external (i.e. institutional zones of practice). This chapter refers to the dominance of the biomedical model which has traditionally influenced case conceptualisation and case formulation to strengths-based perspectives. Contemporary insights to supporting trainees navigate the interplay between individual, relational and societal are explored.

In *Chap. 7,* I distinguish between case management and presenting problem management to provide practical skills to facilitate trainees' competence in the different zones of practice.

In *Chap. 8, Contemporary Areas for Clinical Supervision Integration,* the focus is on addressing contemporary realities. The author discusses key areas identified in contemporary practice with a view to empowering supervisees. The areas include managing culture-bound syndrome, crisis intervention, telepsychology, phototherapy, facilitating client career transitions and a strengths-based approach to case management and conceptualisation are also explored.

In *Chap. 9, Towards Well-being: Self-Care in the Supervisory Space,* Professor Catharina Guse shares her expertise from her several years of both lecturing and professional programme coordination as well her experience as practitioner and researcher in the field of Positive Psychology interventions and wellbeing to inform the critical area of *"Towards Well-being: Self-care in the Supervisory Space".* Strategies for health care professionals and well as clinical supervisors in self-care and self-management are discussed.

In *Chap. 10, Integration of Chapters: Applying a Systemic Lens to Clinical Supervision,* the author integrates the different levels that inform clinical supervision. Implications of the utility of the ecological, relational model in strengthening the lens of trainees to support practising ethically, confidently and innovatively, while also being systematic and clinical are elaborated.

## 1.2   Background: Contextualising Institutions of Practice

**Abstract**  In this chapter, the focus is on contextualising different institutions of practice of health professionals are confronted by. The author locates different 'zones' of practice as Zone A – Institutions of Higher Learning and Zone B – The Health care system. In this chapter, the focus is on highlighting the dynamics, complexities and opportunities for developing resilience that health professionals are confronted by in the provision of mental health care services at institutions.

**Keywords**  Student counselling unit, Health care settings, Preventative, Subjective well-being, Resilience

## 1.3   Practice Zone A (Institutions of Higher Education – Student Counselling Services)

Most higher education institutions in the democratic South Africa are seen as multicultural, multiracial and multilingual. There is diversity in race, culture, language and socio-economic status. Some challenges in South African higher education include high dropout rates, poor career decision-making, a lack of belonging and poor decision-making skills. South Africa also has a high prevalence of social problems that are often carried over by students from a diversity of backgrounds. Research among South African university students indicates they experience high levels of psychosocial vulnerability that can have a direct impact on their academic success (Van Breda, 2013; Wade, 2009; McGowan & Kagee, 2013). In relation to personal challenges faced by students, McGowan and Kagee (2013) investigated the lifetime exposure of 1 337 students at a residential South African university to a range of traumatic life events. The vast majority in this study (90%) reported experiencing at least one of the traumas, with exposure to the suicide or homicide of a close friend or family member being the most frequent (43%). A fifth of the students indicated that the traumas occurred while they were a student.

Student Counselling has been identified to be critical to the academic endeavour of a tertiary institution. Voelker (2003) indicates that more university students may need treatment for depression at a time when colleges and universities do not have the resources to meet that need. She contends that university life coincides with the peak of the onset of mental health symptoms in the general population. It is therefore imperative for higher education institutions to have the facilities to deal with mental health issues.

Alongside the institutional challenges and pressures Psychologists employed in higher education have to contend with, Psychologists also experience many unique challenges with the work context, such as vicarious trauma (Johnson et al., 2011; Maltzman, 2011), suicide ideation (Johnson & Barnett, 2011), burnout (Bradly et al., 2012), discouragement, depression, anxiety, disrupted relationships (Johnson & Barnett, 2011), demanding work, isolation (Webb, 2011), emotional distress (Malinowski, 2013) and alcohol and substance abuse (Smith & Moss, 2009). Barrington and Shakespeare-Finch (2013), however, highlight that although the work that psychologists do is regarded as inherently difficult it 'can provide an opportunity to flourish and grow in ways that few other professions allow' (Barrington & Shakespeare-Finch, 2013, p. 103).

Botha et al. (2005) refer to the increase in demands on Student Counselling and Development (SCD) services and regarded this as problematic in view of limited resources. SCD services are therefore increasingly becoming under pressure to 'do more with less'. In the context of South Africa, this is especially pertinent since the involvement of many South African higher education institutions have been involved in institutional mergers. While there have been benefits for students and institutions from these processes, for many institutions it has translated into additional pressures in terms of physical space, operational budgets, equipment and human resources. Given that it is unlikely that more institutional resources would be made available, the challenge of the creation of additional job resources is therefore left to the creativity of SCD staff and their managers (De Jager, 2012). De Jager (2012) identify that one way of dealing with this challenge is through exploring ways of enhancing staff capacity. To supplement the existing human resource component, reference is made to the role of paid and unpaid interns and enhancing their capacity, through providing relevant training and supervision to navigate and manage contemporary pressures and challenges. The role of SCD services historically was primarily, if not exclusively regarded as a reactive and remedial service with a pathogenic focus. In recent times however, there has been a shift towards a more balanced approach with a focus on more proactive, preventative and constructivist efforts that allow for intervention at the various multisystemic and ecological levels of influence. The need for an integrative framework that integrates the multiple levels that influence health professionals' identity, through the supervisory process is thus required and advocated for in this book.

## 1.4   Practice Zone B: The Health Care System

Health care professionals' practice occurs against the backdrop of various infra-structural challenges in the twenty-first century. In South Africa, mental health practice and care is seen to occur at three levels in the public health system. The primary level consists of community clinics in which social workers and nurses consult on a daily basis but doctors and psychologists only consult once or twice per week (Visagie & Schneider, 2014). At the primary level, psychologists will assess patients and refer them to the other levels if need be. The secondary level has more special-ised services and doctors are always present to present services (Visagie & Schneider, 2014). If there are severe psychological issues, patients will be referred to the tertiary level which is highly specialised. Arcot (2015), however, indicates that while the system sounds great in theory, the implementation has not been as effective as hoped. The services are often seen to be overcrowded and patients who have severe pathology and other issue encounter a long waiting list. Additionally, patients may need to be referred to three doctors just to get medication or see the appropriate specialist which is inefficient and time-consuming (Lund et al., 2010). Challenges facing the health care system in South Africa include an unequal distri-bution of resources, management and leadership crisis, an increased disease burden, pull and push factors and slow progress in restructuring the health care system.

The phenomena of work-related stress and professional burnout have become increasingly recognised in recent health literature and professional contexts (Howard, 2008). In a review of studies on UK Clinical psychologists, Hanningan et al. (2004) concluded that the majority find their work demanding and stress pro-voking. Factors related to levels of burnout included total hours worked, administra-tive/paperwork hours, managed care patient percentage, negative patient behaviours, over involvement with patients and low perceptions of work setting control and lower direct pay percentage (Rupert & Morgan, 2005). Other factors identified to influence the stress experienced in the mental health workplace include increasing complexity and size of caseloads for practitioners. Problems in the workplace such as understaffing and job insecurity, poor job design and lack of a supportive line manager have all been associated with stress in this occupational group (Burrows & McGrath, 2000). In the South, profession-specific difficulties, compounded by the difficult   socio-economic   situation   (Kagee,   2014),   including   violence, communicable disease, urbanisation, civil strife, poverty, sexual violence and abuse, may impact the well-being of psychologists. Jordaan et al. (2007) found that 56.3% of SA psychologists reported symptoms of anxiety and 54.2% reported symptoms of depression.

Limited attention has been paid to the quality of life that psychologists and related health professionals experience at work. In the field of occupational health, however, positive psychologists have explored how the conditions of both the workplace/organisation and the worker can contribute not only to the prevention of stress and ill health but to the promotion of psychological well-being (Schaufeli & Bakker, 2004). Psychologist's overall well-being is regarded as fundamental to their own functioning and the well-being of their clients and patients. Researchers have argued that, if psychologists do not experience high levels of well-being, termed flourishing by Keyes (2005), then problems within the work context and other contexts may adversely impact the quality of their service of clients and patients. Studies over the past two decades have investigated concepts that promote well-being such as a sense of coherence, resilience or personal hardiness, job control, work engagement and flow (May et al., 2004).

## 1.5   Shift Towards Positive Mental Health and Subjective Well-being

Ultimately psychologists as providers of care in the South African health sector must make the commitment suggested by Keyes (2010, p. 26), namely that 'if we want better mental health, we must focus on positive mental health'. One of the key functions of clinical supervision as practised by health professionals such as psychologists includes the restoration of well-being, but there are few guidelines in the supervision literature on how to go about this. Research into concepts from the field of positive psychology such as *work engagement, sense of coherence, self-efficacy, flow and resilience* has begun to provide a detailed understanding of workers' happiness, health and betterment.

*Sense of Coherence*

Antonovsky (1987) proposed that a 'sense of coherence' (SOC) is crucial to the prevention of ill health and consists of three components:

1. Comprehensiveness – characterises how people perceive external events (e.g. what happens to them or around them at work), and how they interpret them. It is the extent to which a person's experience is understandable and predictable to them.
2. Manageability – is the expectation that an individual has adequate resources available to cope with a variety of demands
3. Meaningfulness – is related to emotions and motivation about work, the value an individual gives to a work goal or purpose, in relation to one's own ideals and standards. A lack of meaningfulness can lead to alienation or disengagement from work.

SOC is seen as a relatively stable dispositional personality orientation, which develops early in one's work experiences (Feldt, 2004).

### 1.5.1   Work Engagement

Refers to the extent to which an individual feels positive, involved and fulfilled at work. It is also negatively related to job burnout and is viewed as a useful concept in the management of supervisee stress in a context of 'inherently difficult work'.

### 1.5.2   Self-Efficacy

Refers to one's judgment of one's ability to carry out required tasks, actions and roles. It is also linked to well-being at work. Weak self-efficacy beliefs result in increased levels of burnout and poor performance and the importance of efficacy beliefs in the process of supervision is seen as critical.

### 1.5.3   Flow

The concept of 'flow' has become popularised in recent times and was originally conceptualised by Csikszentmihalyi (1990). Experiencing a flow of work was seen to be referring to having a 'short-term peak experience that is characterised by absorption, work environment and intrinsic motivation' (Bakker, 2004, p. 52). Bakker (2004) referred to supervisory coaching as having a positive relationship on the experience of flow.

### 1.5.4   Resilience

Resilience is referred to as the 'capacity to withstand exceptional stresses and demands without developing stress-related problems' (Carr, 2004, cited in Rothman, 2004). Interventions aimed at promoting resilience could include developing an individual's resources and skills. The practice of supervision is seen to offer a vehicle to build resilience in significant ways.

In this publication, concepts that promote well-being are referred to as most relevant and the reader is invited to reflect on such concepts in informing an ecological framework to strengthen the well-being lens for clinical supervision of health professionals navigating twenty-first-century realities. Reference is also made to a dedicated chapter on self-care and functioning (see Chap. 9, by Professor Tharina

Guse) focuses on strategies that Health Professionals could engage in promoting their well-being. Integrating this aspect into the framework aims to provide possible directions for supervision interventions that go beyond providing traditional 'stand-alone' practices of self-care and stress management strategies and seek to extend the well-being of supervisees.

# References

Antonovsky, A. (1987). *Unraveling the mystery of health. How people manage stress and stay well.* Jossey-Bass.

Arcot, R. (2015). "The traumatic state of psychology: An investigation of the challenges psychologists face when aiming to help trauma survivors in post-apartheid South Africa" (2015). Independent Study Project (ISP) Collection. 2042. https://digitalcollections.sit.edu/isp_collection/2042

Bakker, A. B. (2004). Flow among music teachers and their students: The crossover of peak experiences. *Journal of Vocational Behaviour, 66,* 26–44.

Barrington, A. J., & Shakespeare-Finch, J. (2013). Working with refugee survivors of torture and trauma: An opportunity for vicarious post-traumatic growth. *Counselling Psychology Quarterly, 26*(1), 89–105. https://doi.org/10.1080/15325024.2012.714210

Botha, H. L., Brand, H. J., Cilliers, C. D., Davidov, A., de Jager, A. C., & Smith, D. (2005). The need for and relevance of student counselling and development services in higher education institutions in South Africa. *South African Journal for Higher Education, 19*(1), 73 88.

Bradly, S., Drapeau, M., & Destefano, J. (2012). The relationship between continuing education and perceived competence, professional support and professional value among Clinical Psychologists. *The Journal of Continuing Education in the Health Professions, 32*(1), 31–38.

Burrows, G. D., & McGrath, C. (2000). Stress and mental health professionals. *Stress Medicine, 16,* 269–270.

Carr, A. (2004). Thematic review of family therapy journals 2003. *Journal of Family Therapy, 26,* 429–444.

Csikszentmihalyi, M. (1990). Flow: The psychology of optimal experience. New York: Harper.

De Jager, A. C. (2012). Historical overview. In L. Beekman., C. Cillers., A. C. D. De Jager (Eds.) *Student Counselling and development: Contemporary issues in the Southern African Context* (pp.3–16). Pretoria: UNISA press.

Falender, C. A., & Shafranske, E. P. (2017). *Supervision essentials for the practice of competency-based supervision.* American Psychological association. https://doi.org/10.1037/15962-000

Feldt, T. (2004). Sense of coherence and work characteristics. A cross-lagged structured equation model among managers. *Journal of Occupational and Organisational Psychology, 77,* 323–342.

Hanningan, B., Edwards, D., & Bernard, P. (2004). Stress and stress mangement in clinical psychology. Findings from a systematic review. *Journal of Mental Health, 13,* 235–245.

Howard, F., (2008). Managing stress or ehancing wellbeing? Positive psycholgy's contributions to clinical supervision. *Austrailian Psychologist, 43*(2), 105–113.

Johnson, W. B., & Barnett, J. E. (2011). Preventing problems of professional competence in the face of life-threatening illness. *Professional Psychology: Research and Practice, 42,* 285–293. https://doi.org/10.1037/a0024433

Johnson, W. B., Johnson, S. J., Sullivan, G. R., Bongar, B., Miller, L., & Sammons, M. T. (2011). Psychology in extremis: Preventing problems of professional competence in 75 dangerous practice settings. *Professional Psychology: Research and Practice, 42*(1), 94–104. https://doi.org/10.1037/a0022365

Jordaan, I., Spangenberg, J. J., Watson, M. B., & Fouchè, P. (2007). Emotional stress and coping strategies in South African clinical and counselling psychologists. *South African Journal of Psychology/SuidAfrikaanse Tydskrif vir Sielkunde, 37*, 835–855.

Kagee, A. (2014). South African psychology after 20 years of democracy: Criticality, social development, and relevance. *South African Journal of Psychology/Suid-Afrikaanse Tydskrif vir Sielkunde, 44*, 350–363.

Keyes, C. L. M. (2005). Mental illness and/or mental health? Investigating axioms of the complete state model of health. *Journal of Consulting Clinical Psychology, 73*(3), 539–548.

Keyes, C. L., Dhingra, S. S., & Simoes, E. J. (2010). Change in level of positive mental health as a predictor of future risk of mental illness. *American Journal of Public Health, 100*, 2366–2371. [PMC free article] [PubMed] [Google Scholar].

Lund, C., Kleintjes, S., Kakuma, R., & Flisher, A. J. (2010). Public sector mental health systems in South Africa: Interprovincial comparisons and policy implications. *Social Psychiatry and Psychiatric Epidemiology, 45*, 393404. https://doi.org/10.1007/s00127-009-0078-5

Malinowski, A. J. (2013). Characteristics of job burnout and humor among psychologists. *Humor, 26*(1), 117–133. https://doi.org/10.1515/humor-2013-0007

Maltzman, S. (2011). An organisational self-care model: Practical suggestions for development and implementation. *The Counselling Psychologist, 39*(2), 303–319.

May, D. R., Gilson, R. L., & Harter, L. M. (2004). The psychological conditions of meaningfulness, safety and availability and the engagement of the human spirit at work. [Article]. *Journal of Occupational and Organizational Psychology, 77*, 11–37.

McGowan, T. C., & Kagee, A. (2013). Exposure to traumatic events and symptoms of posttraumatic stress among South African university students. *South African Journal of Psychology, 43*(3), 327–339.

Rupert, P. A., & Morgan, D. J. (2005). Work setting and burnout among professional psychologists. *Professional Psychology: Research and Practice, 36*(5), 544–550. https://doi.org/10.1037/0735-7028.36.5.544

Schaufeli, W. B., & Bakker, A. B. (2004). Job demands, job resources, and their relationship with burnout and engagement: A multi-sample study. *Journal of Organizational Behavior, 25*, 293–315.

Smith, P. L., & Moss, S. B. (2009). Psychologist impairment: What is it, how can it be prevented, and what can be done to address it? *Clinical Psychology: Science and Practice, 16*, 1–15. https://doi.org/10.1111/j.14682850.2009.01137.x

Van Breda, A. D. (2013). Psychosocial vulnerability of social work students. *Social Work Practitioner Researcher, 25*(1), 19–35.

Visagie, S., & Schneider, M. (2014). Implementation of the principles of primary health care in a rural area of South Africa. *African Journal of Primary Health Care Family Medicine, 6*(1), 1–10.

Voelker, R. (2003). Mounting student depression taxing campus mental health services. *Journal of American Medical Association, 289*, 2055–2056. https://doi.org/10.1001/jama.289.16.2055

Wade, B. L. (2009). UNISA social work students' experiences of trauma: An exploratory study from a person-centred perspective. Doctoral Thesis, University of South Africa.

Webb, K. B. (2011). Care of others and self: A suicidal patient's impact on the psychologist. *Professional Psychology: Research and Practice, 42*(3), 215–221. https://doi.org/10.1037/a0022752

# Chapter 2
# The Evolution of Supervisory Models

## 2.1 The Evolution of Supervisory Models: Brief Defining Features

A 'Supervision Model' is defined as the systematic manner in which supervision is applied (Borders et al., 1991). A great number of models have been developed (Gonsalvez & Calvert, 2014). In this chapter, the reader is provided with a brief introduction on the main models. In this chapter, the reader is invited to reflect on how these models have evolved and focus on the relevance of systemic, ecological models in the twenty-first century (Table 2.1).

## 2.2 Relevance of a Systems Perspective in the South African Context

In this publication, we focus on systemic, ecological models of clinical supervision as recent developments in supervision are increasingly becoming informed by such frameworks. In the United States and Canada, supervisors are increasingly supervising therapists (including interns) who have a solid foundation in systemic therapy (Smith, 2009). The importance of supervisors no longer have the luxury of basing their supervision solely on their preferred therapy models, their favourite methods of supervision, the type of supervision relationships they are most comfortable with having, or their personal style (among others).

Many psychologists find the perspective useful for conceptualising the cultural features of clients' lives, their own lives and the treatment process itself. Systems thinking also has been associated as a paradigm that psychologists find useful for shifting focus from an exclusively individual framework to a broader understanding of clients (and helpers) embedded in communities and cultures. This perspective is

K. V. Rawatlal, *Clinical Supervision in South Africa*, SpringerBriefs in Psychology, https://doi.org/10.1007/978-3-031-41929-4_2

**Table 2.1** The evolution of Supervisory Models

| | |
|---|---|
| **The Psychoanalytic/ Psychotherapy model** | This model emerged in the 1920s, with the fundamental belief that supervisees learn best if they experience the qualities of therapy in the supervisory relationship (Bernard & Goodyear, 1992). Smith (2009) indicates that Psychodynamic supervision draws on the clinical data inherent to that theoretical orientation (e.g., affective reactions, defence mechanisms, transference and countertransference, etc.). |
| **Feminist Model of Supervision** | Feminist theory affirms that the personal is political, that is, an individual's experiences are reflective of society's institutionalised attitudes and values (Feminist Therapy Institute, 1999). The Ethical Guidelines for Feminist Therapists (Feminist Therapy Institute, 1999) emphasises the need for therapists to acknowledge power differential in the client-counsellor relationship and work to model the effective use of personal, structural and institutional power. The supervisor-supervisee relationship strives to be egalitarian to the extent possible, with the supervisor maintaining focus on the empowerment of the supervisee. |
| **Cognitive- Behavioural Supervision** | Cognitive-Behavioural supervision makes use of observable cognitions and behaviours – particularly of the supervisee's professional identity and his/ her reaction to the client (Hayes et al., 2003). Cognitive behavioural techniques used in supervision include setting an agenda for supervision sessions, bridging from previous sessions, assigning homework to the supervisee and capsule summaries by the supervisor (Liese & Beck, 1997) |
| **Person-Centred Supervision** | Person-centred supervision assumes that the supervisee has the resources to effectively develop as a counsellor. The supervisor is not seen as an expert in this model, but rather serves as a 'collaborator' with the supervisee. The supervisor's role is to provide an environment in which the supervisee can be open to his/her experience and fully engaged with the client (Lambers, 2000). |
| **Integrative Models of Supervision** | Given the large number of theories and methods that exist with respect to supervision, an infinite number of 'integrations' are seen as possible. In fact, because most counsellors today practice what they describe as integrative counselling, integrative models of supervision are also widely practised (Haynes et al., 2003). |
| **Bernard's Discrimination Model** | Is seen as one of the most commonly used and research integrative models of supervision originally published by Janine Bernard in 1979. This model is comprised of 3 separate foci for supervision (i.e. intervention, conceptualisation and personalisation) and 3 possible supervisor roles (i.e. teacher, counsellor and consultant) (Bernard & Goodyear, 2009). The supervisor could, at any given moment, respond from one of nine ways (three roles x three foci). |
| **Systems Approach** | In the systems approach to supervision, the heart of supervision is the relationship between supervisor and supervisee, which is mutually involving (Holloway, 1995). Holloway (1995) describes seven dimensions of supervision, all connected by the central supervisory relationship. These dimensions include: the functions of supervision, the tasks of supervision, the client, the trainee, the supervisor and the institution (Holloway, 1995). The function and tasks of supervision are at the foreground of interaction, while the latter four dimensions represent unique contextual factors that are, according to Holloway (1995), covert influences in the supervisory process. Supervision is thus seen to be reflective of a unique combination of these seven dimensions. |

(continued)

**Table 2.1** (continued)

| Competency-Based Models | Competency-based models centre around competencies (Falender & Shafranske, 2007), are transtheoretical molecular and start with the 'end in mind'/benchmarks (Gonsalvez & Calvert, 2014). This approach is metatheoretical where clinical competencies are identified in terms of skills, knowledge and attitudes; learning strategies and evaluation procedures are developed; and competency standards, as per criterion references competence consistent with evidence-based practices, and the requirements of the clinical setting, are met (Falender & Shafranske, 2007). |
|---|---|

most relevant in developing contexts such as South Africa which is regarded as a culturally complex and diverse country. South Africa has at least 13 different cultural groups and 11 official languages with population groups designated as Black-Zulu, Coloured (mixed racial ancestry), Indian and White-Afrikaans. Contemporary South Africa is still known for the large economic, racial and cultural differences among groups. This diversity is also reflected in higher education institutions (Nel et al., 2015).

The need for a systemic and integrated approach, which also includes holistic, contextual, local and African indigenous perspectives, is thus highlighted. According to Edwards (2010, 2011) in the South African context, one essential function of psychology institutions is to harmonise old and new, African, Eastern and Western forms of psychological knowledge and activities.

From an integral perspective, psychology includes the study of the structures, states, modes, developmental, behavioural and relational aspects of consciousness, their manifestations in behaviour, and their application for improving humanity in particular and the universe in general (Wilber, 2000). A limited intention of this presentation is to encourage professional and student psychologists to explore their conscious and unconscious experiences towards improved insights and actions in South African and international psychological research and practice. For millennia the perennial philosophy of the great major wisdom and/or spiritual traditions, including ancestor reverence, Judaism, Hinduism, Buddhism, Taoism, Christianity and Islam, recognised a holistic form of psychology that included different levels of consciousness, from subconscious to self-conscious and beyond (Assagioli, 2012; Aurobindo, 2011; Huxley, 1946; Mutwa, 2003; Wilber, 2000). For example, ancestral consciousness recognises recently departed ancestors, especially those remembered with reverence. Hinduism refers to the dance of Shiva. Although not systematised and labelled as such, in prevalence, effect and function, such holistic, spiritual, communal psychology still remains predominant in the developing regions and countries of planet earth including most of Southern Africa (Edwards, 2011). This calls for an integral as well as local approach, which is the central theme in this contribution.

In South Africa, it is seen as imperative that Psychologists possess indigenous knowledge and skills as opposed to exposure to only Western training models as South Africa, with its host of cultural groups and languages, is known for its diversity. Most of these models, in an African context, have often been found to be inappropriate and not useful (Olivier, 1992; Seedat et al., 2001). Criticisms levelled against Psychology and the institutions responsible for training psychologists in South Africa, is that they turn a deaf ear towards knowledge systems that are rooted in the historical and experiential realities of the indigenous people (Chitindingu & Mkhize, 2016).

# References

Assagioli, R. (2012). *Psychosynthesis. A collection of basic writings*. The Synthesis Centre.

Aurobindo, S. (2011). *The integral yoga*. Lotus Press.

Bernard, J. M., & Goodyear, R. K. (1992). *Fundamentals of clinical supervision* (1st ed.). Allyn & Bacon.

Bernard, J.M., & Goodyear, R.K. (2009). *Fundamentals of clinical supervision* (4th ed.). Needham Heights, MA: Allyn & Bacon.

Borders, L. D., Bernard, J. M., Dye, H. A., Fong, M. L., Henderson, P., & Nance, D. W. (1991). Curriculum guide for training counselor supervisors: Rationale, development, and implementation. *Counselor Education and Supervision, 31*, 58–80.

Chitindingu, E., & Mkhize, N. (2016). Listening to Black African psychologists' experiences of social and academic inclusion: Incorporating indigenous knowledge systems into the curriculum. *Alternation Journal, 18*, 72–98. Retrieved from https://journals.ukzn.ac.za/index.php/soa/article/view/1355

Edwards, S. D. (2010). An overview of the University of Zululand community psychology project. *University of Zululand Journal of Psychology, 25*(1), 3–20.

Edwards, S. D. (2011). A psychology of indigenous healing in Southern Africa. *Journal of Psychology in Africa, 21*(3), 335–347.

Falender, C. A., & Shafranske, E. P. (2007). Competence in competency-based supervision practice: Construct and application. *Professional Psychology: Research and Practice, 38*, 232–240. https://doi.org/10.1037/0735-7028.38.3.232

Feminist Therapy Institute. (1999). *Feminist therapy code of ethics*. Retrieved August 14, 2009, from http://www.feminist-therapy-institute.org/ethics.html

Gonsalvez, C. J., & Calvert, F. L. (2014). Competency-based models of supervision: Principles and applications, promises and challenges. *Australian Psychologist, 49*, 200–208. https://doi.org/10.1111/ap.12055

Hayes, R., Corey, G., & Moulton, P. (2003). *Clinical Supervision in the Health Professions: A Practical Guide*. Pacific Grove, CA: Brooks/Cole.

Haynes, R., Corey, G., & Moulton, P. (2003). *Clinical supervision in the helping professions: A practical guide*. Brooks/Cole.

Holloway, E. (1995). *Clinical supervision: A systems approach*. Sage.

Huxley, A. (1946). *The perennial philosophy*. Fontana.

Lambers, E. (2000). Supervision in person-centered therapy: Facilitating congruence. In E. Mearns & B. Thorne (Eds.), *Person-centered therapy today: New frontiers in theory and practice* (pp. 196–211). Sage.

Liese, B. S., & Beck, J. S. (1997). Cognitive therapy supervision. In C. E. Watkins Jr. (Ed.), *Handbook of psychotherapy supervision* (pp. 114–133). Wiley.

Mutwa, V. C. (2003). *Zulu shaman. Dreams, prophecies and mysteries*. Destiny Books.

Nel, N., Nel, J. A., Adams B. G., & De Beer L. T. (2015). Assessing cultural intelligence, personality and identity amongst young white Afrikaans-speaking students: A preliminary study. *South African Journal of Human Resource Management, 13*, 1–12. https://doi.org/10.4102/sajhrm.v13i1.643

Olivier, L. (1992). The need for counselling in South Africa. In J. Uys (Ed.), *Psychological counselling in the South African context* (pp. 14–33). Maskew Miller Longman.

Seedat, M., Duncan, N., & Lazarus, S. (2001). Community psychology: Theory, method, and practice. In M. Seedat, N. Duncan, & S. Lazarus (Eds.), *Community psychology: Theory, method, and practice* (pp. 1–14). Cape Town.

Smith, K. (2009). *A brief summary of supervision models*. [ebook] pp. 1–10. Available at: https://www.marquette.edu/education/.../brief-summary-of-supervision-models.pdf. Accessed 4 Apr 2019.

Wilber, K. (2000). *Integral psychology*. Shambhala.

# Chapter 3
# Towards a Systemic and Relational Ecological Framework to Clinical Supervision

## 3.1 The Ecological Framework

Since Bronfenbrenner popularised ecological models in developmental psychology nearly 25 years ago (e.g. Bronfenbrenner, 1979), there has been a growing interest in ecological or contextual frameworks in psychology. While Bronfenbrenner's (1979) model has been elaborated on, given its developmental focus, there is a wide assortment of theories aligned to the ecological perspective from a variety of disciplines and subdisciplines, including health promotion, health psychology, developmental psychology and community psychology. In addition, some counselling psychology programs have adopted an ecological framework as their training model, such as the program at the University of Oregon (McWhirter et al., 2001). In this publication, given the development focus of an ecological perspective, the author promotes an elaboration of the framework to include clinical supervision of developing health professionals.

The subsystems that influence human development are now unpacked. Bronfenbrenner (1979) suggests that the ecology of human development is the process of mutual accommodation between the person and the environment. Using this ecological perspective and drawing from a model developed by the Pan American Health Organisation for changing youth behaviour (Breinbauer & Maddaleno, 2005), Petersen et al. (2011) adapted the framework for guiding the development and implementation of mental health promotion and prevention programmes in scarce resource contexts. I further discuss (Fig. 3.1) how the framework will be expanded for the purposes of this text through presenting a phased and structured approach that incorporates the various subsystems known to influence human development. This framework is indicated to lay the foundation for providing a systemic and structured approach to clinical supervision (Table 3.1).

© The Author(s), under exclusive license to Springer Nature Switzerland AG 2023
K. V. Rawatlal, *Clinical Supervision in South Africa*, SpringerBriefs in Psychology,
https://doi.org/10.1007/978-3-031-41929-4_3

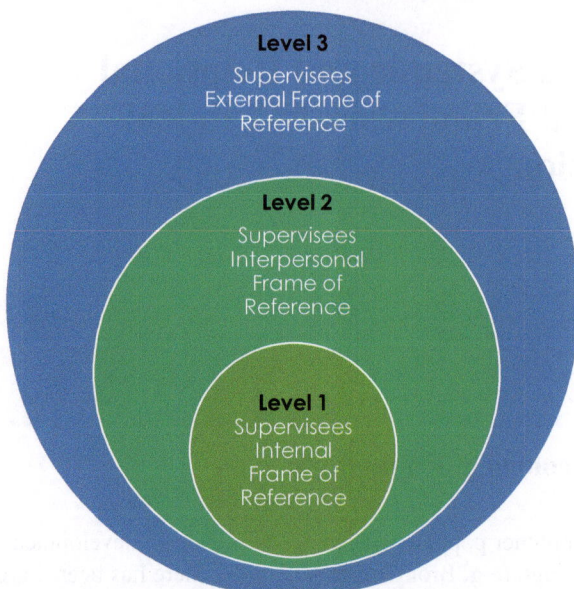

**Fig. 3.1** An ecological framework applied to clinical supervision

**Table 3.1** Ecological framework of human development

| Levels of influence | Intervening with the different levels |
|---|---|
| Individual level theories | Aimed at strengthening the personal influences or assets that a person brings to a situation, such as coping skills, cognitive abilities, beliefs and motivations. Interventions are also aimed at reducing the impact of emotional trauma and strengthening self-regulation and resilience ability. At this level, there is a focus on strengthening the self-efficacy of a person |
| Interpersonal level theories | Aimed at strengthening the protective influence of interpersonal relationships and strengthening the social support that occurs within the person's microsystem or immediate surroundings |
| Community level theories | Aimed at the person's relationship with public, private, organisations or institutions, the broad social setting in which relationships occur, the institutional policies and regulations |

## 3.2   Ecological Framework Applied to Clinical Supervision

Using the previous conceptualisations and adaptations of Bronfenbrenner's (1979) ecological model, the author presents an ecological model to clinical supervision. In addition to primarily focusing on the dynamics that strengthen the different sub-systems (e.g. wellbeing perspective, positive psychology, integrating indigenous knowledge systems, supervision and training issues), this framework differs from purist ecological/contextual models of clinical supervision in 2 ways.

1. Consistent with emerging trends in the area, the individual or person is incorporated as a system in this framework. Characteristics of individuals (e.g. cultural beliefs, personality, life experiences, etc.) play necessary roles in determining how one interacts with, adjusts to and manages working with clients/patients from different and similar contexts.

2. Navigating social structures of different institutions that health professionals practice is highlighted. Classical ecological models are seen to delimit the macrosystem to consist of values. In this publication, the macrosystem is broadened to include the structure of economic status, race, culture and gender. The assumption underlying this decision is that we live in a society that is stratified across a variety of demographic, social location and identity. This is also consistent with many social inequality psychology scholars (Olivier, 1992; Seedat et al., 2001; Edwards, 2010; Chitindingu & Mkhize, 2016) who argue in favour of addressing indigenous, marginalised and nondominant groups in training models. In the explication of the model, the author discusses the role of the clinical supervisor in supporting trainees in navigating the dialectical relationship between values and social structures to better manage client and patient presentations. In Fig. 3.1, an ecological framework of clinical supervision for health professionals is presented.

## 3.2.1 Level One: Supervisee's Internal Frame of Reference

At this level, the focus in Clinical Supervision is aimed at identifying the personal characteristics, the identity trainees have developed in relation to the communities and cultural and healing practices that shape their thinking. The clinical supervision process thus provides the space for exploring motivation, beliefs strengthening the personal influences or assets that a person brings to a situation, such as coping skills, cognitive abilities, beliefs and motivations. At the individual level, clinical supervisors may explore with trainee health professionals; identity and purpose, personal characteristics they possess as trainees, adaptability, the stress response and coping and leadership and life skills. Level one is expanded in Chap. 4.

## 3.2.2 Level Two: Supervisee's Interpersonal Frame of Reference

At this level, the focus is on the supervisee's clinical supervision encounter/experience/consultation with the clinical supervisor. This places emphasis on the supervisor's competence in providing a relevant, positive and high-quality supervisory relationship that enables supervisee's social responsibility as a health professional to navigate twenty-first century realities. The focus is on developing supervisee's competence to engage in reflective practice, adopting a positive psychology lens (incorporating strengths-based and resilience competence). At level two, I also address supervisors serving as role models and their identification as 'cultural selves'. This is also introduced to address the need in the South African context to provide post-colonial and resilience-based supervision. Level two is expanded in Chap. 5.

### 3.2.3    Level Three: Navigating the External (The Institutional, Organisational, Societal setting)

At this level, the role of the clinical supervisor in supporting supervisees navigate institutional/organisational contexts/systems/environment is emphasised. The context that the socio-ecological model provides the supervisee and supervisor a structured way of intervening that not only addresses the individual level but also the various sub-systems that influence. This level also discusses the influence of institutional challenges such as resource allocation, economic conditions, policies and regulations that influence the professional identity and practice of health professionals at different institutions. Level three is expanded in Chap. 6.

## References

Breinbauer, C., & Maddaleno, M. (2005). *Youth: Choices and change: Promoting healthy behaviours in adolescents*. Pan American Health Organisation.

Bronfenbrenner, U. (1979). *The ecology of human development: Experiments by nature and design*. Harvard University Press.

Chitindingu, E., & Mkhize, N. (2016). Listening to Black African psychologists' experiences of social and academic inclusion: Incorporating indigenous knowledge systems into the curriculum. *Alternation Journal, 18*, 72–98.

Edwards, S. D. (2010). An overview of the University of Zululand community psychology project. *University of Zululand Journal of Psychology, 25*(1), 3–20.

McWhirter, B. T., McWhirter, E. H., Flojo, J. R., Torres, D. M. & Gragg, K. M. (2001). Ecological training model: University of Oregon. Presentation at the 4th National Counseling Psychology Conference, Houston, TX.

Olivier, L. (1992). The need for counselling in South Africa. In J. Uys (Ed.), *Psychological counselling in the South African context* (pp. 14–33). Maskew Miller Longman.

Petersen, I., Bhana, A., Flisher, A., Swartz, L., & Richter, L. (2011). *Promoting mental health in scarce-resource contexts: emerging evidence and practice*. University of Cape Town.

Seedat, M., Duncan, N., & Lazarus, S. (2001). Community psychology: Theory, method, and practice. In M. Seedat, N. Duncan, & S. Lazarus (Eds.), *Community psychology: Theory, method, and practice* (pp. 1–14). Cape Town.

# Chapter 4
# Level One (The Core) Informing Supervisee's Internal Lens of Reference

## 4.1 Level 1: Supervisee's Internal Frame of Reference

### 4.1.1 Introduction

In the field of Counselling Psychology, many theories emphasise self-awareness as an essential part of psychological health (Corey, 2001; Critelli, 1987; Hamachek, 1992; Schneider-Corey & Corey, 2002). As a Counselling Psychologist involved in managing the training programme and coordinating the practicum module (clinical supervision of supervisees), my experience suggests that many supervisees commence their graduate training programme not prepared for this personal focus. Many trainees expect their training to emphasise assessment and intervention strategies, psychopathology and treatment. While these areas represent significant aspects of counsellor education, the importance of personal awareness should not be overlooked (Myers, 2003). It is this sense of lack of personal or self-awareness that is seen to define the level of professionalism that health professionals practice with.

'Professionalism' has been referred to as being under increasing scrutiny across the health and social care professions with many of the issues that emerge later in health professional careers being linked to a broad range of behaviours distinct from their technical ability (Professionalism in Healthcare Professionals, 2014). These behaviours include increased reports of inappropriate or unprofessional behaviour, and increased numbers of 'fitness to practice' cases heard by the Health Professionals Council. For example, the Health Professions Council of South Africa (HPCSA) report of ethical misconduct cases by registered psychologists in South Africa during the period 2007–2013 indicated that 'at the turn of the century, there has been a change and increase in ethical transgressions that include sexual or dual relationships with patients as well as unprofessional, unethical or negligent practice (Nortje & Hoffmann, 2015).

© The Author(s), under exclusive license to Springer Nature Switzerland AG 2023
K. V. Rawatlal, *Clinical Supervision in South Africa*, SpringerBriefs in Psychology,
https://doi.org/10.1007/978-3-031-41929-4_4

Also linked to the implications of a lack of self-awareness and professionalism is the impact on health professionals in experiencing compassion fatigue. Compassion fatigue has been identified to be one of the biggest health problems facing mental health practitioners with close to 50% of practitioners being at risk of this phenomenon (Injeyan et al., 2011).

### 4.1.2  Addressing the Core (Individual Level)

In this chapter, the focus is on trainees (supervisees) strengthening the core level or individual level. Supporting trainees being 'in touch' with their life's core personal struggles (core issues and derivatives, vulnerabilities) facilitates trainees empathising with and gaining insight into client/patient's struggles, and with the challenges they face in overcoming the obstacles. The focus is on developing health professionals' self-awareness as an integral component of their professional training and clinical supervision.

Emphasis is placed in clinical supervision on supervisees engaging in

- Self-assessment and monitoring of their strengths and personality areas for development
- Identification of predisposing thinking patterns about self that either enhance or that may serve to deter their practice as health professionals
- Exploration of motives
- Their identity, beliefs and positionality based on their own cultural awareness and world views

Theodore Reik (1948) spoke in the 1940s about listening with the 'third ear', a form of self-awareness through which therapists can be sensitive to and aware of what patients *communicate* through therapists' *inner experience of their own person* while engaged in the therapeutic process with the patient-meaning that this *third ear* 'listens' to the patient by expanding their listening to include therapists' own inner experiences and reactions to patients/clients.

### 4.1.3  Self-Awareness and Cultural Awareness

While personal therapy has always been promoted as an important aspect of counsellor training, efforts to determine the relationship between personal therapy and counsellor effectiveness have been inconclusive (Macran & Shapiro, 1998; Macran et al., 1999; McEwen & Duncan, 1993). Myers (2003) study supported the view that while therapy is certainly one way towards self-awareness, it is not the only way. Self-awareness refers to the understanding of a person's personal thoughts, beliefs, feelings, behaviours and attitudes (Tyson, 2007). Other authors have also highlighted that without a complete understanding of the self, there is also a limited chance that an individual will be open to learning about another culture or multiple cultures (Furness, 2005). The American Psychological Association (APA, 2003) multicultural guidelines encourage clinicians to 'recognise that, as cultural beings, they may hold beliefs and attitudes that can detrimentally influence their perceptions and interactions with individuals who are ethically and racially different from themselves' (p. 382). Developing self-awareness is thus seen as paramount to preventing clinicians' biases from impeding how they serve culturally different clients.

Strategies to develop cultural awareness

- Encouraging the supervisee to understand the clients' cultural identity
- During clinical supervision, the supervisor can ask the supervisee to reflect on any instances where there are conflicts between cultures which might result in barriers to therapy
- In a broader sense, supervisees could also be encouraged to create training material and online training involving issues of diversity, cultural awareness and cultural assessment

### 4.1.4   Worldviews

In this section, the focus is the importance of exploring worldviews in strengthening the individual level competencies and resilience of practitioners. By exposing students to the concept of *worldviews* early in their training, clinical supervisors can better meet professionalism mandates related to self-awareness, bias and bolster the status of the social and behavioural sciences (Tilburt et al., 2007). *Worldview* refers to ' a philosophy of life that answers all the most fundamental questions of human existence' (Nicholi, 2004). Derived from the German term *weltanschauung* (meaning the 'view of the world'), worldview is a way of naming the life perspective on which one approaches problems, looks for solutions, and thinks about life options. If students do not reflect both on the assumptions they bring to their training and also on the assumptions of the biomedical worldview, they may not gain sufficient insight into the biases that influence their professional development (Tilburt et al., 2007). Without self-reflection, students risk 'getting into trouble' – as Mark Twain warned-by steadfastly adhering to only one worldview without acknowledging that there are others, or by being unable to reconcile various worldviews when they interact (or collide) (Tilburt et al., 2007).

### 4.1.5   Motivation

Beatty (2012) indicates that there is merit in including some consideration of motives as part of the training process. According to Hlot and Luborsky's (1958) study (cited by Narcross & Farbar, 2005), psychotherapists frequently report that they only recognise the reasons they choose their discipline well into their career or during the course of intensive personal therapy. Further, Beatty (2012) indicates that it seems incongruous that an exploration of motives would be omitted from the training process, given the emphasis on self-development and self-awareness. Beatty (2012) extends that the adage that a counsellor can only take the client as far as they have themselves have gone in terms of self-exploration seems to confirm, if only on an anecdotal level, that by neglecting such as important aspect on one's journey, they may neglect a similarly important element of that of a client's (Beatty, 2012).

Further reference is also made to the importance of incorporating this aspect. For a profession that has been so concerned with the genesis of human behaviour and emotion and the unconscious it is surprising that more attention is not paid to what draws people to a career described by Freud (1937) as the 'impossible profession' (cited by Bager-Charlson, 2010). As Sussman (1995) points out, psychotherapy has a lot to say about the 'unconscious factors in the choice of an occupation' (quoted by Bager-Charlson, 2010, p.13) and yet, it would appear, very little to say about those which motivates its own practitioners. The dearth of discussion on this topic within the available research and within training programmes indicates that is an area that could benefit wider consideration for strengthening the profession.

### 4.1.6 Identity as a Professional

In this domain, it is highlighted that there exists another level to professionalism, related more to 'Identity as a Professional'. This level is recognised as the individual's perception of themselves as professionals. Practitioners' views of where professionalism comes from identify two main sources of influence: the first, the respondents' personal qualities and the second, the context of the immediate situation. Many health professionals felt that professionalism was a consequence of qualities that the individuals brought to the profession – perhaps not actually innate but certainly preexisting. A common theme was that the 'right sort of person' will be attracted to a profession, for example, a caring person will be attracted to a caring profession. Researchers have also found that students had similar personality profiles to those on the 'big five personality dimension, extraversion, conscientiousness, neuroticism'. While professionalism was seen as rooted in personal values and beliefs, becoming a fully-fledged professional was seen as a 'work in progress' (Table 4.1).

**Table 4.1** Key domains informing the core

| Self-Awareness and Cultural Awareness | Worldview |
|---|---|
| Identification and monitoring of strengths, personality developmental areas, thinking patterns, resistance, defence mechanisms, transference and countertransference issues. Understanding self as emerging from different cultural groups, core beliefs and the shaping of identity. | Supervisee's identification of his or her life perspective to understand approaching problems, identification of solutions, and thinking about life options. This may also be influenced by culture. |
| Motivation | Identity as a Professional |
| Identification and timeous reflection of factors that motivate supervisees to pursue a career as a health professional is seen to promote a 'state of subjective well-being' and resilience. Motivation is thus seen as a crucial, internal asset to the strengthening of professional identity. | In this domain, supervisees identify and reflect on how their values, sense of morality and well-being have evolved in their sense of identity as a professional. Supervisees also reflect on how their individual profile is aligned with the personality profile of a health professional. |

# References

American Psychological Association. (2003). Guidelines on multicultural education, training, research, practice, and organizational change for psychologists. *American Psychologist, 58*, 377–402.

Bager-Charlson, S. (2010). *Why therapists choose to become therapists*. Karnac Books.

Beatty, E. (2012). *A study of motivations amongst contemporary trainee counsellors for pursuing a career in Psychotherapy*. Unpublished dissertation. Dublin Business School (DBS). Retrieved from https://esource.dbs.ie › ba_beatty_e_2012

Corey, G. (2001). *Theory and practice of counseling and psychotherapy*. Brooks/Cole.

Critelli, J. (1987). *Personal grovvth and effective behavior*. Holt.

Furness, S. (2005). Shifting sands: Developing cultural competence. *Practice, 17*, 247–256. https://doi.org/10.1080/09503150500425638

Hamachek, D. (1992). *Encounters with the self*. Harcourt Brace Jovanovich College Publishers.

Holt, R. R., & Luborsky, L. (1958). *Personality patterns of psychiatrists: A study of methods for selecting residents* (Vol. 1). Basic Books.

Injeyan, M. C., Shuman, C., Shugar, A., Chitayat, D., Atenafu, E. G., & Kaiser, A. (2011). Personality traitsassociated with genetic counselor compassion fatigue: The roles of dispositional optimism and locus of control. *Journal of Genetic Counseling, 20*, 526540. https://doi.org/10.1007/s10897-011-9379-4

Macran, S., & Shapiro, D. (1998). The role of personal therapy for therapists: A review. *British Journal of Medical Psychology, 7. (1)*, 13–25.

Macran, S., Stiles, W., & Smith, J. (1999). How does personal therapy affect therapists' practice? Journal of. *Counseling Psychology, 4 6(4), 4 1*, 9–43.

McEwen, J., & Duncan, P. (1993). Personal therapy in the training of psychologists. *Canadian Psychology, 3 4(2),* l 86-197.

Myers, S. (2003). Reflections on reflecting: How self-awareness promotes personal growth. *The Person-Centred Journal, 10.*

Nicholi, A. M., Jr. (2004). Introduction: Definition and significance of a worldview. In A. M. Josephson & J. R. Peteet (Eds.), *Handbook of spirituality and worldview in clinical practice* (pp. 3–12). American Psychiatric Publishing Inc..

Norcross, J. C., & Farber, B. A. (2005). Choosing psychotherapy as a career: Beyond "I want to help people". *Journal of Clinical Psychology, 61*(8), 939–943. https://doi.org/10.1002/jclp.20175

Nortje, N., & Hoffmann, W. A. (2015). Ethical misconduct by registered psychologists in South Africa during the period 2007–2013. *South African Journal of Psychology, 45*(2), 260–270. https://doi.org/10.1177/0081246315571194

Professionalism in healthcare professionals. (2014). Health and Care Professions Council ((HCPC). Parkhouse, London. Retrieved from https://www.hcpc-uk.org/globalassets/resources/reports/professionalism-in-healthcare-professionals.pdf

Reik, T. (1983). *Listening with the third ear: The inner experience of a psychoanalyst book description* (3rd ed.). Published by Farrar, Straus and Giroux Rinehart and Winston Inc..

Schneider-Corey, M., & Corey, G. (2002). *Croups: Process and practice*. Brooks/Cole.

Sussman, M. B. (1995). *A perilous calling: The hazards of psychotherapy practice*. Wiley.

Tilburt, J., Ford, J. G., Howerton, M. W., Gary, T. L., Lai, G. Y., Bolen, S., Baffi, C., Wilson, R. F., Tanpitukpongse, T. P., Powe, N. R., Bass, E. B., & Sugarman, J. (2007). *Clinical Trials, 4*(3), 264–269. https://doi.org/10.1177/1740774507079440. PMID: 17715253.

Tyson, S. Y. (2007). Can cultural competence be achieved without attending to racism? *Issues in Mental Health Nursing, 28*(12), 1341–1344.

# Chapter 5
# Supervisee's Interpersonal Frame of Reference

## 5.1 Level 2 – Supervisee's Interpersonal Frame of Reference

In this chapter, the focus is on strengthening supervisee's external (supervisee and supervisor relationship) frame of reference. The focus is on the role of the supervisor to serve as a role model/mentor to enhance supervisee's capacity for self-reflection and reflective ability, provision of strengths-based clinical supervision and clinical supervision for addressing diversity and multi-culturalism.

## 5.2 Self-Reflection

The purpose of self-reflection is to promote supervisee's self-awareness and potential for personal change. Reflection is referred to involve a number of skills (such as observation, self-awareness, critical thinking, self-evaluation and receiving others' perspectives) and has the outcome of integrating this understanding into future planning and goal setting (Mann et al., 2009). Student practitioners or supervisees are less able to reflect-in-action than more experienced practitioners (Mann et al., 2009). They need more structure to support deep reflection on their experiences and this draws the focus to the role of the supervisee's relationship with the supervisor.

### 5.2.1 The Process of Reflection

Carroll (2009a, b) introduced a systematic process of reflection and the author presents an adapted version. Supervisees and supervisors can use Table 5.1 not only as a model for focusing on reflective practice, but also as a schemata that supports the

© The Author(s), under exclusive license to Springer Nature Switzerland AG 2023
K. V. Rawatlal, *Clinical Supervision in South Africa*, SpringerBriefs in Psychology,
https://doi.org/10.1007/978-3-031-41929-4_5

**Table 5.1** Initiating Clinical Supervision and structuring the reflective process

| Preparing for reflection | Reflective process | Action following reflection |
|---|---|---|
| **Step 1: Supervisor reflects on the core** (supervisee has assessed their individual personality strengths, motivation world view, beliefs), the supervise is ready to shift to Level 2 | Event/s Situations: Allowing the reflective process to be felt and experienced | Supervisee transfers learning to work (practical knowing), integrates new learning with existing knowledge |
| **Step 2: PREPARING THE ENVIRONMENT:** The supervisee presents the client/patient presenting problem and the results of a Mental Status Examination (MSE) of the client/patient. The supervisor provides a containing physical, emotional and psychological space that also conveys respect for cultural issues and issues of diversity | Supervisor assists the supervisee recall/describe/give attention to and focus | Other possibilities: Letting come: reinterpretation. New perspectives widen openness to new information and meanings |
| **Step 3: Preparing the Reflective Relationship** The focus is on dialogue, engagement, establishing the supervisory experience as a collaborative space for supervisee's development and growth. Client management and case management is explored | Stay with emotional reaction: allow confusion, disorientation and monitor blocks | Articulation of learning |
| **Step 4: Preparing Myself** Supervisees to explore their motivation, the importance of reflection, consequences of not reflecting. Being able to communicate with supervisee without feeling threatened and punitively evaluated | Analysis and meaning making: careful consideration. Resonating what I intuitively feel, think and sense | |

Stages of reflection, adapted from Carroll (2009a, b)

reader step back and look at the process by which reflection takes place – reflection on reflection. According to Carroll (2009a, b), the meta-cognition involved here moves from a focus on experience itself to a focus on the experience of reflection in order to review its effectiveness.

**Preparing for Reflection** Highlights the relationship/s that surround the supervisory, counselling, or coaching relationship. How power may be used in this relationship, the kind of engagement involved and the type of conversation used, all contribute to reflection. Ability to monitor motivation and adapting to a non-judgemental stance is seen to further support the reflective process.

**The reflective process (attention)**

Siegel (2007) divides attention into three parts:

*Alerting* – involving attention, vigilance and alertness
*Orienting* – selecting certain information from a variety of options to scan or select
*Executive attention* – our attention to sift and control the process…what happened…describe the event…don't evaluate it

**Action following reflection**

This step involves integrating and making sense of what supervisee and supervisor have focused on and integrating new learning with existing knowledge as reflected in the figure.

## 5.3   Internal Supervisor

Casement (1985) developed the idea that an 'internal supervisor' guides the supervisee to reflect upon the meaning of their communication and therapeutic progress. Internal supervisor highlights that as we engage with our work, we become our own supervisor, monitoring, thinking, evaluating, and assessing what is going on. An important part of internal supervision is 'trial identifying' with the patient. This refers to the supervisee putting themselves in the position of the client/patient in order to monitor their role in the clinical process, considering how the client/patient maybe experiencing supervisees input in the session. Another part of the internal supervisor is for the supervisee to look for unconscious prompts from the patient/client that can help supervisee recognise when a patient/client is being affected by supervisee in ways that were not intended or anticipated. The development of an internal supervisor remains underdeveloped, however as experience grows, the supervisee's internal locus of evaluation (Villas-Boas Bowen, 1986) grows with her/him, and the supervisee develops his own internal supervisor (Rønnestad & Skovholt, 2003). Rønnestad and Skovholt (2003) thus highlight the need for existing models of supervision to evolve into a more-encompassing internal supervisor model.

## 5.3.1   Towards a 'Resilience-Based' Mindset in Approaching Supervisees

In empowering supervisees to navigate the systemic and contextual realities discussed in the different practice zones (Chap. 1), it is important for supervisees to be reflective of the evolution of counselling and supervision relationships.

Reference is made to the previous dominance of Eurocentric, individualistic psychological theories and practices that emerged from colonisation (Hernández & McDowell, 2010; Hernández-Wolfe, 2011). Colonisation is identified in the literature as a process of systemic suppression of the beliefs, values and practices of subordinated cultural groups to champion that of the dominant Western European groups (Hernández & McDowell, 2010; Hernández-Wolfe, 2011). The critical postcolonial and resilience based approaches seek to develop new frameworks that acknowledge a diversity of experience and integrate multiple ways of knowing and attention to cultural diversity (Butler-Byrd, 2010; Hernández & McDowell, 2010; Reynaga-Abiko, 2010; Singh & Chun, 2010). The relevance of this focus is that it acknowledges the influence of social context and power structures in developing and maintaining emotional distress, it recognises that supervisees and clients are multifaceted, intersectional and embedded in their context/s rather than within compartmentalised identities (Hernández & McDowell, 2010; Porter & Vasquez, 1997; Singh & Chun, 2010). With a focus on resilience, attention is drawn to marginalised individual's ability to rebound and rise above challenging experiences rooted in oppression (Singh & Chun, 2010).

## 5.4   In Practice

In reference to integrating a 'resilience-based' approach, supervisors are invited to reflect on what this might involve in practice. The following listed below may enhance this process for supervisors:

• Supervisors can honour diverse cultural backgrounds by practising cultural humility, developing knowledge regarding socio-political and historical contexts, and engaging in holistic approaches to healing (Butler-Byrd, 2010) (See also Chap. 8 in which I include questions that can inform trainees in developing cultural knowledge).
• Supervision from a critical postcolonial-ad resilience-based model is also said to further the clinical development of both the supervisee and the supervisor by engaging in an analysis of the influence of power and oppression in both the therapeutic and supervisory encounters (Hernández & McDowell, 2010; Singh & Chun, 2010).
• This practice in supervision supports trainees develop critical consciousness, enhances their sense of empowerment and renders the supervisor and supervisee

accountable to help begin in addressing the inequities that influence client distress Butler-Byrd, 2010; Hernández & McDowell, 2010).

- Supervisors can serve as role models by bringing their own cultural selves in supervisory discussions through power sharing experience. As Ramírez Stege et al. (2019) indicate that rather than having supervisors prove cultural competence to supervisees of colour, both supervisor and supervisee are engaged in a *continual dialogue* and experiential practice of positioning their cultural selves in the supervisory dyads.

In further developing trainees' reflective ability, the importance of reflective inventories, keeping a diary or journaling is also emphasised. Keeping a diary, or journalling is often mentioned in the literature (e.g. Chirema, 2007; Hiemestra, 2001; Phipps, 2005). It is identified as a way of looking back at experiences in detail to learn from them and adjust future behaviour of trainees. Specific prompts or cues (usually a series of questions) can support the practitioner or student to move from describing experiences to analysing, making meaning and setting goals for the future (e.g. Boud & Walker, 1998; Findlay et al., 2011; Freeman, 2001; Roberts, 2009).

In reflection in the clinical encounter, student practitioners are less able to reflect-in-action than more experienced practitioners (Mann et al., 2009) and need more structure to support deep reflection on their experiences. Lewis (2013) and students developed a series of scaffolding questions (Fig. 5.1) to support students' ability to answer the clinical educator's question 'how did that session go?' Students use this series of questions to reflect on their clinical experiences (whether an assessment, intervention or consultation), making brief notes before then discussing with their clinical educator or peers. These questions could also be used and adapted by trainee practitioners to support their reflections with their clinical supervisor. The author presents an adapted list of questions based on Lewis (2013) initial questions.

- What did you notice about yourself prior to the session?
- What did you notice about self during the session (transference and countertransference)?
- What did you notice about self-post the session?

**Were your goals for the session achieved?**

- 3 things that went well and why.
- 3 things that didn't go well and why.

**Reflection in relation to your client**

- Were your goals for the session achieved?
- What improvements were built on from previous feedback?
- How would you describe the client's experience of the session?
- What do you need to find out before the next session?

(Information, evidence)
*What could you aim for in the next session in the light of today's performance?

| Preparing for Reflection | Reflective Process | Action following reflection |
| --- | --- | --- |

**Preparing for Reflection**

•**Step 1: Supervisor reflects on the core** (supervisee has assessed their individual personality strenghts, motivation world view, beliefs), the supervise is ready to shift to Level 2

•**Step 2: PREPARING THE ENVIRONMENT:The** supervisee presents the client/patients presenting problem and the results of a Mental Status Examination (MSE) of the client/patient. The supervisor provides a containing physical, emotional and psychological space that also conveys respect for cultural issues and issues of diversity

•**Step 3: Preparing the Reflective Relationship** The focus is on dialogue, engagement, establishing the supervisory experience as a collaborative space for supervisees development and growth. Client management and case manahement is explored

•**Step 4: Preparing Myself** Supervisees to explore their motivation, the importance of reflection, consequences of not reflecting. Being able to communicate with superivisee without feeling threated and punitively evaluated

**Reflective Process**

•Event/s Situations: Allowing the reflective process to be felt and experienced

•Supervisor assist the supervisee recall/describe/give attention to and focus

•Stay with emotional reaction: allow confusion, disorientation and monitor blocks

•Analyis and meaning making: careful consideration.

• Resonating what i intuitively feel, think and sense

**Action following reflection**

•Supervisee transfers learning to work (practical knowing), integrates new learning with existing knowledge

•Other possibilitues: Letting come: reinterpretation. New perspectives widen openess to new information and meanings

•Articulation of learning

**Fig. 5.1** Reflection after a clinical encounter. (Adapted from Lewis, 2013)

### Reflection in relation to your own performance

• How did you feel in the session?
• Compare your performance with the client's performance and participation.
• What would you improve for the next session?

# References

Boud, D., & Walker, D. (1998). Promoting reflection in professional courses: the challenge of context. *Studies in Higher Education, 23*(2), 191–206.

Butler-Byrd, N. M. (2010). An African American supervisor's reflections on multicultural supervision. *Training and Education in Professional Psychology, 4*, 11–15. https://doi.org/10.1037/a0018351

Carroll, M. (2009a). From mindless to mindful practice: On learning reflection in supervision. *Australian Journal of Psychotherapy, 15*(4), 38–49.

Carroll, M. (2009b). Supervision: Critical reflection for transformational learning, part 1. *The Clinical Supervisor, 28*(2), 210–220.

Casement, P. J. (1985). The internal supervisor. In *P.J. Casement on learning from the patient*. Tavistock Publications.

Chirema, K. (2007). The use of reflective journals in the promotion of reflection and learning in post-registration nursing students. *Nurse Education Today, 27*(3), 192–202.

Findlay, N., Dempsey, S., & Warren-Forward, H. (2011). Development and validation of reflective inventories: assisting radiation therapists with reflective practice. *Journal of Radiotherapy in Practice, 10*(1), 3–12.

Freeman, M. (2001). Reflective logs: An aid to clinical teaching and learning. *International Journal of Language and Communication Disorders, 36* (2 Supplement), 411–416.

Hernández, P., & McDowell, T. (2010). Intersectionality, power, and relational safety in context: Key concepts in clinical supervision. *Training and Education in Professional Psychology, 4*, 29–35. https://doi.org/10.1037/a0017064

Hernández-Wolfe, P. (2011). Decolonization and "mental" health: A Mestiza's journey in the borderlands. *Women & Therapy, 34*, 293–306. https://doi.org/10.1080/02703149.2011.580687

Hiemestra, R. (2001). Uses and benefits of journal writing. In English, L.M. and Gillen, M.A. (Eds), Promoting Journal Writing in Adult Education. *New Directions in Adult and Continuing Education, 90*, 19–26.

Lewis, A. (2013). Reflective practice what is it and how do I do it? *Journal of Clinical Practice in Speech-Language Pathology, 15*(2), 70–73.

Mann, K., Gordon, J., & MacLeod, A. (2009). Reflection and reflective practice in health professions education: A systematic review. *Advances in Health Sciences Education, 14*(4), 595–621.

Phipps, J. (2005). E-journaling: achieving interactive education online. *Educause Quarterly, 28*(1), 62–65.

Porter, N., & Vasquez, M. (1997). Covision: Feminist supervision, process, and collaboration. In J. Worell & N. G. Johnson (Eds.), *Shaping the future of feminist psychology: Education, research, and practice* (pp. 155–171). American Psychological Association Press. https://doi.org/10.1037/10245-007

Ramírez Stege, A. M., Chin, M. Y., & Graham, S. R. (2019, September 16). A critical postcolonial and resilience-based framework of supervision in action. *Training and Education in Professional Psychology*. https://doi.org/10.1037/tep0000276. Advance online publication.

Reynaga-Abiko, G. (2010). Opportunity amidst challenge: Reflections of a Latina supervisor. *Training and Education in Professional Psychology, 4*, 19–25. https://doi.org/10.1037/a0017052

Roberts, A. (2009). Encouraging reflective practice in periods of professional workplace experience: the development of a conceptual model. *Reflective Practice, 10*(5), 633–644.

Rønnestad, M. H., & Skovholt, T. M. (2003). The journey of the counselor and therapist: Research findings and perspectives on professional development. *Journal of Career Development, 30*, 5–44.

Singh, A., & Chun, K. Y. S. (2010). "From the margins to the center": Moving towards a resilience-based model of supervision for queer people of color supervisors. *Training and Education in Professional Psychology, 4*, 36–46. https://doi.org/10.1037/a0017373

Villas-Boas Bowen, M. C. (1986). Personality differences and person centered supervision. *Person-Centered Review, 1*, 291–309.

# Chapter 6
# Navigating the External (Institutional)

## 6.1 Navigating the External (Institutions of Practice)

At both sites (higher education and the health care system), historically services were primarily if not exclusively regarded as reactive and remedial service with a pathogenic focus. In recent years, there has been a shift towards a more balanced approach with a focus on more proactive, preventative and constructivist efforts that allow for intervention at the various multisystemic and ecological levels of influence.

Student counsellor roles and functions have expanded significantly to include more proactive, preventative and developmental intervention. Core services identified by the Southern African Association for Counselling and Development in Higher education include individual and group counselling and psychotherapy, career assessments and counselling, as well as academic and personal skills development (de jager, 2012). Additional student counsellor functions include student advocacy, faculty consultation, networking, collaboration and professional training and development of interns and staff (de Jager, 2012). The influence of the medical model on student counselling practice has been noted (e.g. Beamish, 2005; Kadambi et al., 2010; Lafollette, 2009; Stone & Archer, 1990). This model has been associated with psychology's propensity to adopt a pathological approach to psychological functioning, viewing it in terms of the presence or absence of psychopathology (Naidoo, 2001). The permeation of this model into student counselling seems related to a perceived increase in severe psychopathology amongst university and college students in the United States (e.g. Beamish, 2005; Kadambi et al., 2010; Lafolette, 2009; Stone & Archer, 1990).

In the health care system, advances in the biomedical and the behavioural sciences have paved the way for the integration of medical practice towards the biopsychosocial approach. Thus, dealing with health and illness overtakes looking for the presence or absence of the disease (the biomedical paradigm) to the biopsychosocial paradigm in which health means a state of complete physical, psychological

© The Author(s), under exclusive license to Springer Nature Switzerland AG 2023
K. V. Rawatlal, *Clinical Supervision in South Africa*, SpringerBriefs in Psychology,
https://doi.org/10.1007/978-3-031-41929-4_6

and social well-being. The clinical role of psychologists as health providers is seen as diverse with the varying areas of caregiving (primary, secondary and tertiary care) and a variety of subspecialities.

The development and evaluation of psychological interventions from a positive psychological perspective has gained momentum in the last 5 years. Joseph and Linley (2005) have indicated that a positive psychological perspective is relevant in all therapeutic contexts and that the role of psychologists should go beyond alleviating distress to facilitating well-being and fulfilment as this could serve as a buffer against the development of psychopathology. In integrating a positive psychology lens to clinical supervision, I also make reference to recent literature that highlights the need for a shift in thinking about case formulation. Traditionally case formulation has been associated with identification of deficits. A 'best practice' formulation draws attention to the service user's resources and strengths in surviving what are nearly always challenging life situations. Formulation can be defined as the process of co-constructing a hypothesis or 'best guess' about the origins of a person's difficulties in the context of their relationships, social circumstances, life events and the sense they have made of them. It is seen to provide a structure for thinking together with the client of the service provider about how to understand their experiences and how to move forward. Formulation thus draws on two equally important sources of evidence: the clinician brings knowledge derived from theory, research and clinical experience, while the service user brings expertise about their own life and the meaning and impact of their relationships and circumstance. In this way, formulation is 'the tool used by clinicians to relate theory to practice' (Butler, 2008, p. 2) (Fig. 6.1).

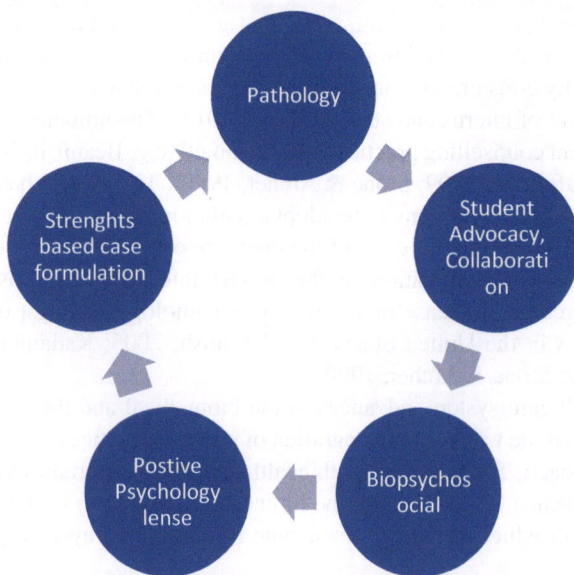

**Fig. 6.1** The evolution in the zones of practice

## 6.2 Practice Issues

In supporting supervisees manage patients/clients, the author later (Chap. 7) differentiates between client/patient presentation management and case management. In navigating the external, the focus is also on Integrating a positive psychology lens in therapeutic intervention of patient/client work. The focus is also on integrating a formulation-based perspective. From this perspective, the notion that the work of every mental health professional, whatever their training, should be based on the principle: that however unusual, confusing, risky, destructive, overwhelming, or frightening someone's thoughts, feelings and behaviours are, there is a way of making sense of them is supported (Johnstone, 2018). The central task of mental health professionals is to work alongside service users to create meaning out of chaos and despair and formulation is a powerful and effective way of doing this. Best practice formulation is thus regarded as a radical act that restores agency, meaning and hope. It provides a framework for witnessing people's stories, hearing their suffering and space for their voices (Johnstone, 2018).

### 6.2.1 What Is It

Unlike diagnosis, formulation is not about making an expert judgement, nor is it based on deficits. Instead, a best-practice formulation draws attention to the service user's resources and strengths in surviving what are nearly always very challenging life situations.

For these reasons, the DCP Good Practice Guidelines (2011) specify a number of principles in formulating, including that the process should be collaborative, respectful of service users' views about accuracy and helpfulness, expressed in ordinary and accessible language, culturally sensitive, non-judgemental, and inclusive of strengths and achievements (DCP, 2011, pp. 29–30). Psychologists are expected to take a reflective stance that reduces the risk of Johnstone 35 using formulation in insensitive, nonconsenting, or disempowering ways (DCP, 2011, p. 21).

## References

Beamish, P. M. (2005). Introduction to the special section - Severe and persistent mental illness on college campuses: Considerations for service provision. *Journal of College Counseling, 8*(2), 138–139. https://doi.org/10.1002/j.2161-1882.2005.tb00080

De Jager, A. (2012). Historical overview. In L. Beekman, C. Cilliers, & A. de Jager (Eds.), *Student counselling and development: Contemporary issues in the southern African context* (pp. 3–17). Unisa Press.

Division of Clinical Psychology. (2011). *Good practice guidelines on the use of psychological formulation*. British Psychological Society.

Johnstone, L. (2018). Psychological formulation as an alternative to psychiatric diagnosis. *Journal of Humanistic Psychology., 58*(1), 30–46.

Joseph, S. & Linley, P. A. (2005). Positive adjustment to threatening events: An organismic valuing theory of growth through adversity. Review of General Psychology, 9 (3), 262–280. Retrieved from https://doi.org/10.1037/1089-2680.9.3.262.

Kadambi, M., Audet, C. T., & Knish, S. (2010). Counseling higher education students. *Journal of College Student Psychotherapy, 24*(3), 213.

LaFollette, A. M. (2009). The evolution of university counseling: From educational guidance to multicultural competence, severe mental illness and crisis planning. *Graduate Journal of Counseling Psychology, 1*(2), 1–9. Retrieved from http://epublications.marquette.edu/gjcp/vol1/iss2/11

Stone, G. L., & Archer, J. (1990). College and university counseling centers in the 1990s: Challenges and limits. *Counseling Psychologist, 18*, 539–607. https://doi.org/10.1177/0011000090184001

# Chapter 7
# Case Management and Presenting Problem Management

## 7.1 Case Management and Presenting Problem Management

In acknowledging the logistical challenges of practising in resource-constrained contexts (discussed in Chap. 2, practice zone A and B) I differentiate between client/patient presentation management and case management to support supervisees navigate such settings.

### 7.1.1 Case Management

#### 7.1.1.1 Establishing Familiarity at the Clinical Practicum Site

In case management, it is important that the supervisor encourages supervisee to become familiar with the referral or clinical practicum site.

- Identification of the key role players, health professionals, coordinators, administrators, emergency personnel contact details (consider if a Memorandum of Understanding is in place to support the identification and enhance service delivery)
- Identification of the referral pathways and cross-referral pathways that exist at the institution
- Identification of the information data sources (i.e. access to academic records/ patients/clients files)
- Limits to confidentiality and boundaries with respect to other health professionals at the site

© The Author(s), under exclusive license to Springer Nature Switzerland AG 2023  39
K. V. Rawatlal, *Clinical Supervision in South Africa*, SpringerBriefs in Psychology,
https://doi.org/10.1007/978-3-031-41929-4_7

### 7.1.1.2   Preparation for the Session

It is important to review any background information that could support understanding the client/patient's reason for reason and presenting problem

- Peruse previous client/patient file
- Peruse academic records (identify periods where the client's performance declined, reconciled or gained momentum) as this is also related to psychological and emotional state of mind
- Identify previous referral/consultation with health professionals and contact details
- Identify previous medication/prescriptions
- Identify previous recommendations for type of intervention, i.e. Psychotherapy, Psychiatric consult, Medical Consult
- Identity barriers to accessing the services

### 7.1.1.3   Complete Intake Forms

Preceding the session,

- Provides information about the therapeutic process
- Benefits and merits of Psychotherapeutic intervention
- Informed consent, confidentiality, limits to confidentiality
- Structuring of sessions and contracting for sessions
- In the event of an emergency/crisis situation, availability of Psychologist and other contact details
- Implications for mislabelling, misdiagnosing and implications for 'fitness to practice' and reporting thereof
- Client/patient signs the informed consent and confidentiality form/s
- Client/patient completes the intake form (biographical information and presenting problem)
- Client/patient may also be administered a self-report measure such as the BAI or BDI inventory

## *7.1.2   Presenting Problem Management*

In management of the presenting problem and in supporting a shift away from a biomedical, deficit approach that has dominated many practice settings, Smith's (2006) strengths-based counselling model is also incorporated as a resource to navigate practice realities.

**Stage 1: Helping the Patient/Client Tell Their Story (Therapeutic Alliance)**

Task 1: Task one would involve helping the client/patient provide a narrative account as to their reasons for presenting and their timeous presentation. A stance of collaboration is fostered and the intention is for the client/patient to develop insight as to the source of the presenting problem, experience a state of empowerment that they have initiated the contact with the health professional. The supervisee assists the client/patient with verbalising, affirming and validating the experience or the cause for concern. The supervisee provides the space for them to ventilate, release pent up emotions and feelings that render them vulnerable. The use of non-judgemental, open-ended and probing questions supports the client develop rapport and trust. From a strengths-based perspective, the goal is to also support clients/patients understand their personality, explore interpersonal patterns and dimensions. The focus for the supervisee is on identification with source of the problem and the impact on the individual. Supervisees may ask the client/patient to develop a problem list to refine goal setting, which will occur at the next stage IN A CRISIS (see Presenting Problem Management and Crisis Intervention, page 86.). The focus is on evaluating the client's functional ability, pre the session, in the session, and post the session. Questions can be posed to the client regarding their plans for the rest of the day, the next day or questions related to support (family and friends) the client will come in to contact with

**Stage 2: Identifying Strengths**

Task 2: In task two, the Health Professional helps the client/patient identify significant blindspots related to their problems (e.g. patterns of resistance, withdrawal, pessimistic views, overgeneralisation, catastrophising thinking patterns). This may also mean effectively challenging blindspots that facilitates bringing new perspectives to awareness that supports clients think more realistically about problems, opportunities and solutions

**Stage 3: Assessing Presenting Problems**

Task 3: The supervisee assesses areas for intervention at the different levels. This also helps the client/patient develop insight to factors that pose a risk to their growth and development. Supervisee assesses *individual level* (self-esteem issues, motivation, depression/negative schemata/overgeneralisation, rationalising, emotional, labelling behaviour), *the interpersonal level* (self, relationships with others, family) that may perpetuate and maintain unhealthy core beliefs or that may serve as enhancing and positive influences and *community level influences* that influence thinking and patterns of behaviour (see application of the Wellness Wheel by, Rawatlal, K.V.- forthcoming).

**Stage 4: Encouraging and Instilling Hope**

Strengths-based counselling is conceptualised as encouragement counselling that is based on behavioural principles of positive reinforcement. Encouragement has been defined as feedback that emphasises individuals' efforts or improvement rather than the outcomes of their efforts. Psychologists positively reinforce clients for coming to therapy, whether voluntarily or involuntarily, by emphasising their strengths (Dreikurs, 1971).

**Stage 5: Framing Solutions**

The strengths-based therapist understands that you need not solve a problem to find a solution to a troubling situation (Walter & Peller, 1992). A useful counselling technique for this stage is the exception question whereby the psychologist actively looks for exceptions to the occurrence of the problem and enlists clients/patients help in finding practical solutions to the core or presenting problem. Practical solutions may include adopting a different time-management schedule or seeking the help of another health professional. Strengths-based psychologists engage in solution-building conversations with their clients (de Shazer, 1985, 1994). They address how the client is addressing problems rather than the problems themselves (Berg & De Jong, 1996).

**Stage 6: Building Strength and Competence**

At this stage, the reality that people require competence and strength-building across the developmental lifespan is acknowledged. Strengths that might be built during psychotherapy include courage, insight, optimism, perseverance, putting troubles in perspective and finding purpose (Walsh, 2004). During the competence-building stage, therapists help clients learn that they are not powerless to effect change in their lives.

**Stage 7: Empowering**

During empowerment, the practitioner works to develop a critical consciousness about the interconnections in the realities of the client's sociopolitical life (Lee, 2001; Simon, 1990). The practitioner develops conscientization (Bretton, 1993), which examines the inseparability of private troubles and public issues addressed. Empowering counsellors explore the social and cultural origins of the client's actions, and they focus on the context in which clients' problems occurred. Practitioners recognise that problems are not necessarily within the person and that the client has most likely attempted a solution for each problem, with varying degrees of success and failure. The counselling psychologist helps clients activate resources within themselves and their communities (Lee, 2001).

**Stage 8: Changing**

Strengths-based counsellors understand that change is a process, not an isolated event. Throughout counselling, psychologists speak the language of change with their clients (Selekman, 1997). Change is seen to consist of productive dialogue that helps clients become aware of what modifications they must make to improve their lives and to describe what strengths or resources they have to make those. Reframing also assists the process of change as reframing examines a life experience previously viewed as negative and takes a fresh look, describing the experience as positive.

**Stage 9: Building Resilience**

The strength-based psychologist actively seeks to help build resiliency that will fortify them from a recurrence of the same problem or insulate themselves from similar problems (Dunst et al., 1988).

**Stage 10: Evaluating and Terminating**

During this phase, both therapist and client honour the progress that has been made (Weick & Chamberlain, 2002). They determine whether the client has accomplished goals, whether changes can be attributed to the intervention, and what client strengths and environmental resources were most significant in helping them achieve their goals. During termination, strength-based counsellors seek to answer questions such as Has the client accomplished what he or she contracted to do? What factors brought about the client changes? Does the current situation suggest the need for further counselling/intervention.

### 7.1.3   Managing the Interplay Between Individual, Relational, Community and Societal

In drawing attention to preventing the onset of pathology in individual client/patient, it is sometimes necessary for the supervisee to be familiar with how to address multiple levels at the same time. Supervisees need to be trained on how to sustain prevention efforts over time and also achieve population-level impact. The socio-ecological model was created to shift the narrative about mental health and mental illness from an individual issue to include the social and environmental responsibility of others (Biglan et al., 2012). Figure 7.1 depicts a socio-ecological model that considers the complex interplay between individual, relationship, community and societal influences. It allows the therapist to understand the range of factors that clients/patients need to navigate to promote their wellness.

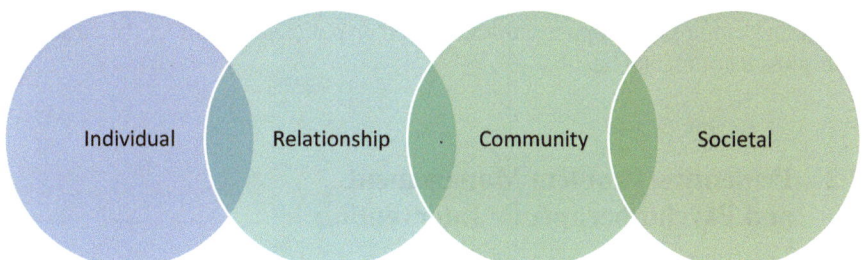

**Fig. 7.1**  The interplay between individual, relationship, community and societal influences

**Individual Level Influences**

The first level identifies biological and personal history factors that increase the likelihood of developing a mental health disorder. Some of the factors may include age, education, income, substance use, or history of abuse. Prevention efforts at this level include changes in thinking patterns, attitudes, beliefs, and behaviours. Specific approaches may include brief solution-focused intervention, stress management, conflict resolution, life skills training, socio-emotional learning and relationships skills programs.

**Relationship Level Influences**

The second level examines patients/clients close relationships that may increase the risk of developing a mental health disorder or condition. Dynamics to be explored include the influence of the family, peer norms and social norms that either hamper or promote healthy relationships.

**Community Level Influences**

The third level explores the settings such as schools, workplaces, and neighbourhoods, in which social relationships occur and seeks to identify the characteristics of these settings that are associated with developing a mental health disorder or condition. Prevention strategies at this level may focus on improving the physical and social environment in these settings (e.g. by creating safe places where people live, learn, work, and play) and by addressing other conditions that give rise to developing mental health problems in communities (e.g. neighbourhood poverty, residential segregation, instability, high density of alcohol outlets, unemployment).

**Societal Level Influences**

The fourth level looks at the broad societal factor that helps create a climate, e.g. a climate which violence or gangsterism is encouraged or inhibited. These factors include social and cultural norms that support violence as an acceptable way to resolve conflicts. Other large societal factors include health, economic, educational and social policies that help to maintain economic or social inequalities between groups in society. Prevention strategies at this level include efforts to promote or challenge societal norms or core beliefs that either strengthen or weaken mental health well-being as well as efforts to strengthen household financial security, education and employment opportunities, and other policies that affect the structural determinants of mental health.

## 7.2   Presenting Problem Management and Psychotherapeutic Intervention

*Psychological counselling* is defined by the British Association for Counselling (BAC, 1989, 1992) as the professional use, regulated by principles of a relationship, in which the client is helped to acquire a better knowledge of himself/herself and of his/her own emotional problems, and to sustain his/her emotional growth and the optimal development of his/her own resources. The counselling relationship may change on the basis of the client's needs, but it concerns essentially developmental tasks and it aims at:

– Working out specific problems
– Taking decisions
– Facing episodes of crisis
– Developing personal insights and a better self-knowledge
– Elaborate the feelings linked to one's personal conflicts
– Improving interpersonal relationships

Further characteristics that define counselling intervention are:

– An explicit request by the client
– The setting
– The adoption of a theoretical frame by the counsellor

The next intervention on the continuum is *psychotherapy,* which aims at purposes of change and cure of individuals and requires a different professional training. Practicing without a theoretical framework will render practitioners vulnerable and directionless while being bombarded by hundreds of impressions and pieces of information in every therapeutic session. While having a foundational understanding, that combines both theory and practice of the different psychotherapeutic modalities is important, supervisees also need to adopt a critical psychology lens. This lens supports supervisees adapt their methods to best fit the public sector and address intervening with a diversity of clients with limited access to resources (Smith, 2013). Smith (2013) calls for a shift in the thinking of universities and professionals in different practice settings, to how psychotherapists will adapt to these new demands.

Prilleltensky and Nelson (2002, p. 21) describe psychotherapeutic theories in terms of powerful tools that have both oppressive and emancipatory effects on therapeutic interventions because 'they can portray humans (clients/patients) as active or passive, altruistic or driven to violence'. According to the authors, theories serve 'constraining or emancipatory purposes', and the authors believe that awareness of the oppressive effects of theories should be an integral part of the practice of critical psychology. This view holds much value for supervisees and practitioners in the South African contexts where the application of Western-oriented theories is dominant and there is a need to make psychological treatment more accessible and relevant to the needs of the country.

The author now highlights some of the most popular therapeutic approaches and also briefly includes some of the issues related to application in the different South African settings of practice. As mentioned above, one of the requisites of psychological counselling is the adoption of a theoretical frame of reference. The dominant orientations and their associated operational terms in the field of counselling are now highlighted in Table 7.1.

Foundational Therapeutic Skills to Presenting Problem Management.

**Table 7.1**  Dominant orientations in the field of therapeutic approaches

| CLASSICAL PSYCHOANALYTIC AND PSYCHODYNAMIC THERAPY | COGNITIVE-BEHAVIOURAL THERAPY |
|---|---|
| Psychoanalysis can take a variety of forms that may vary from practitioner to practitioner. Psychoanalysts support the notion that unconscious conflict is at the root of every emotional difficulty (Wolberg, 1982). The unconscious is assessed via dreams, slips of the tongue, post-hypnotic suggestions, analysis of the symbolic content of psychological symptoms or material derived from projective techniques or free association (Corey, 2005). Psychodynamic therapies have many forms of which ego-state (the development of different ego states, e.g.a nurturing ego-state or a victim ego-state), object relations (placing more emphasis on environment than instincts), and interpersonal therapy (such as transactional analysis with child-, adult- and parent ego states) are some (Prochaska and Norcross, 2007, p. 63). in the African context, relational psychoanalysis (Mitchell & Aron, 1999; Mitchell, 2000) is identified as an important intervention. The relational approach recognizes that there is purpose and relevance in things within the consulting room that may initially appear irrational and expressed through ritual, myth, symbol and metaphor. Relational psychoanalysis thus draws attention to the dictates of cultural wisdom and knowledge rather than to unyielding claims of universal scientific 'truth' and claims of an objective authority regarding such truth. The discourse of relational psychoanalysis can encompass the context of culture and meanings given by race, gender, class, and vocabularies of difference and divergence and the intrapsychic is not understood as isolated and independent of the interpersonal (Knight, 2009). The literature identifies many practical and logistical problems making it difficult to conduct long-term psycho-analytic treatment. As psychoanalysis is not a specific treatment modality but a philosophical framework, its theories and techniques can be applied in a range of settings and integrated with the theories and techniques of other approaches (Wedding & Corsini, 2014). | Cognitive behavioural therapy (CBT), Beck (1976) is an insight-oriented modality which focuses on changing negative thoughts and maladaptive beliefs (Corey, 2005). CBT is based on the premise that one's feelings are determined by one's thinking (Prochaska & Norcross, 2007). The goal of CBT is to identify and restructure the clients' automatic thoughts about themselves and others which lead to emotional disturbance. CBT techniques include emotional processing techniques, schema-focused therapy, modifying need for approval (Leahy, 2003), Socratic questioning (Paul & Elder, 2006) and cognitive shifting. CT remains a popular modality for application in different contexts as it provides novice therapists with a systematic and structured way of approaching therapeutic work. It is also regarded as a briefer form on therapy, is time-limited and drives client agency through engagement of activities such as developing a collaborative therapeutic alliance, setting goals and homework activities. Criticisms about CT from a cultural perspective is that 'rational thinking' is a scientific orientation that fits well with the preferred way of thinking of white, male, Europeans and American (Prochaska & Norcross, 2007, p. 345). Young (2009) conducted a systematic review of CT in the literature identified 15 outcome studies, and suggests that cognitive therapy is a viable and much-needed approach in South Africa. Psychologists practising CBT in South concur with Hays (1995) that the approach is transportable to local contexts, although minor adaptations are required at times. Cognitive therapists and their clients should attempt to understand how the context has shaped and continues to shape the client's negative core beliefs, and how these beliefs influence thinking, before arranging interactions with reality that are designed to change unhelpful beliefs. In cultural tailoring of CBT, case conceptualisations and treatment plans should always accommodate clients' cultural models and beliefs (see Rawatlal, K.V, forthcoming). |

**Narrative therapy**

Within a narrative frame, human problems are viewed as arising from and being maintained by oppressive stories which dominate the person's life (Carr, 1998). Human problems occur when the way in which people's lives are storied by themselves and others does not significantly fit with their lived experience. Indeed, significant aspects of their lived experience may contradict the dominant narrative in their lives. Developing therapeutic solutions to problems, within the narrative frame, involves opening space for the authoring of alternative stories, the possibility of which have previously been marginalized by the dominant oppressive narrative which maintains the problem. These alternative stories typically are preferred by clients, fit with, and do not contradict significant aspects of lived experience and open up more possibilities for clients controlling their own lives. The narrative approach rests on the assumption that narratives are not representations of reflections of identities, lives and problems. Rather narratives constitute identities, lives and problems (Bruner, 1986, 1987,1991). According to this position, the process of therapeutic re-authoring personal narratives changes lives, problems and identities because personal narratives are constitutive of identity. The narrative approach to therapy has been used in meaningful ways in a number of countries which are historically embedded in social injustice, violence, and dispossession (Denborough, 2011). Narrative approaches to therapy might offer practitioners diverse and meaningful means of engaging with the profession and their clients. Furthermore, narrative practice's valuing of community, family, relationship and connectedness together with its understanding that identity is relational, relate well to the African philosophy and may thus provide valuable support for the relevance of this approach in South Africa (Smit, 2016).

**Person/client-Centred therapy**

Person-centred therapy focuses on the process of therapy and identifies the conditions that are necessary for a relationship to bring about constructive personality change (Prochaska & Norcross, 2007). Rogers believed in human beings' actualising tendency and that people respond to reality as they experience it (Prochaska & Norcross, 2007). Prochaska and Norcross (2007, p. 162) caution that the preoccupation of Rogers with selfhood, individuation and self-actualisation is culture-specific and that the high value attributed to individualism is more Western and may not be shared by all cultures. Nonetheless, client-centred skills such as empathy, positive regard and genuineness are most crucial in any therapeutic encounter.

(continued)

**Table 7.1** (continued)

| Solutions-focused therapy | Integrative & eclectic therapy |
|---|---|
| Is based on the positive assumptions that individuals are active agents and have the ability to construct solutions that enhance their lives. The therapy is brief and takes place over 6–10 sessions (De Shazer, 1985), and even as few as three sessions (Caon, n.d.). The fundamental concepts of solution-focused therapy are to build on strengths and to speak solution languages (Prochaska & Norcross, 2007). It is based on positive psychology as opposed to a problem focus, and is focused on the future, not the past (Caon, n.d.). | Many therapists admit that they are eclectic in their practice and choose therapies that they believe will work best for a specific client. Eclecticism described by Evans and Gilbert (2009) is seen as a random choice without a particular desire for theoretical coherence. In contrast to eclectic therapies is the integrative model of psychotherapy... which refers to development towards a 'conceptually coherent, principles, theoretical combination of two or more specific approaches' (ibid., 2009). There is, as the name implies, an emphasis on integrating the underlying theories of various psychotherapies along with techniques from each. Another form of integrative therapy is assimilative integration, where therapists use one theoretical orientation as a foundation and incorporate strategies and techniques from other orientations as they progress (Messer, 1992). |

Patient-centred or person-centred principles form the foundation of any therapy and counselling consultation. The following key principles form this foundation:

- The therapist must maintain an empathic stance and understanding of the client/patient
- The therapist must be able to communicate in non-judgemental manner to the client
- The therapist must be genuine and authentic with the client/patient and demonstrate unconditional positive regard for the client/patient
- The client is perceived as resilient, trustworthy, resourceful, self-directed and capable of making constructive changes that will influence their lives positively (adapted from Corey, 2005, p. 164).
- Certain techniques and 'ways of being' with a client that are generic to all therapeutic encounters include attending, listening, understanding, expressing empathy, probing problem areas and summarising the client's current dilemma (Egan, 1998).

Presenting Problem Management and Crisis Intervention

Gilliland and James (1993, p.3) as cited in Beekman et al., 2012, state that crisis is a perception of an event or situation as an intolerable difficulty that exceeds the resources and coping mechanism of an individual'. Health professionals such as Psychologists are often the first point of contact with clients/outpatients in crisis in higher education/institutional/hospital and primary health care settings. Clients/outpatients arrive at the settings in a crisis state and Psychologists are called, both during and after hours, to support them. Patients/Clients in crisis states typically manifest psychological decomposition to a state of anxiety or depression, active suicidal ideation or suicidal behaviour, substance intoxication and psychotic episodes being most prevalent. In addition, psychological sequelae following the death of a significant other, unplanned pregnancies, partner abuse, physical and sexual assault and negative health diagnoses, i.e. HIV/AIDS or cancer, are often the focus of crisis intervention (Beekman et al., 2012).

In South African society, there is also the need to acknowledge patients/clients whose worldviews and belief systems are entrenched in non-Western ideologies and practices. Crisis presentations maybe characterised with experiencing signs and symptoms of 'culture bound" syndrome, whereby the person may present in a state of psychosis, dissociation and altered state of consciousness. Mental health services need to thus embrace spiritual beliefs and address such presentations. The importance of identifying spiritual/traditional healers in the community setting is therefore highlighted in supporting clients/patients in crisis presentations. Indeed, spiritual healers are 'highly respected members of the community and provide great stability' and 'are believed to understand the cultural signs, symptoms, or distress experiences' (Yorke et al., 2016, 174–194; Crawford & Lipsedge, 2004, 131–148). A competent therapist is able to respond to different types of crises through establishing reliable sources of support and strengthening the relationship with referral sources in the settings they may find themselves in. These may extend to include external sources of assistance and support and include traditional healers and other role players who identify clients in crisis such as academic tutors, clinic staff, student representative councils, risk management services and clinic/hospital co-ordinators.

Generic crisis intervention steps are however relevant, and the author presents some of the stages implored in the different contexts she has practised. Some of the steps referred to are also supported by the Crisis intervention models proposed by Gilliland and James (1993) and Bancroft and Graham (1996).

1. *Assess the client/patient's mental, emotional and functional state*: The first stage of crisis intervention involves the assessment of the client's immediate mental and emotional state. This includes an assessment of the client's level of lethality, level of anxiety, degree of agitation and severity of distress. The Psychologist can also assess the client/patient's ability to conduct functional activities such as plan to go to work/class the next day, and activities the client will be performing post the therapy session. It is important for the Psychologist/Health Professional to assess the client's sense of motivation and agency to pursue any of these 'functional' activities to inform whether the client poses a threat to self or others. The client's mental, emotional state and functional state will inform the Psychologist as to whether the client will be responsive to the psychological management/intervention plan or whether the client will require immediate restraint, medical assistance or hospitalisation. In a crisis, presentation is also important to assess the immediate support network/peers/contacts the patient/client will make contact with after the session. In further assessing functioning and making a referral, the practitioner may also conduct the DSM-IV-Global Assessment of Functioning (GAF).

2. *Establishing Safety:* This may need to take place at any stage in the crisis intervention and usually involves making sure the client is no longer at risk of physical harm (physical safety) and feels able to discuss the cause of their distress with the therapist in a confidential place (emotional safety).

3. *Providing support, facilitating the expression of emotion, positive regard, optimism, normalising:* During this stage, the therapist helps the client restore a state of equilibrium and containment (i.e. creating a state of control from the messiness of the crisis) to process the event. Ventilation or release from the pent feelings of the crisis is encouraged through supporting the client verbalise and release the emotions. Common emotional states include helplessness, anger, grief, frustration and guilt. Within the context of therapy, the therapist shares what emotions, feelings are to be expected as normal in the aftermath of the crisis. Psychoeducation on management and further referral for processing is also encouraged.

4. *Exploring alternatives and identifying strengths and opportunities:* A client/patient in distress is often unable to explore options adequately and the therapist may provide suggestions concerning supporting alternatives. If circumstances permit, therapists may also engage the client in brief problem-solving. Overall, establishing alternatives and identifying opportunities helps the client to regain a sense of control over the situation and develop a state of optimism.

5. *Making plans:* It is important to help the client create a state of orderliness through identifying plans and steps to helping them achieve their short-term and long-term goals. Consider somethings that need to them to think practically and matters that they need to follow-up with to reconcile their progress and follow-up in therapy sessions.

6. *Obtaining commitment and reinforcing coping:* During the final stage, clients are asked to summarise their management plan in order to demonstrate that they are responsible for the options that are available to them (see Rawatlal, K.V, forthcoming, Developing a Wellness Plan). A follow-up session can be scheduled.

# References

Bancroft, J., & Graham, C. (1996). Crisis intervention. In S. Bloch (Ed.), *Introduction to the psychotherapies* (3rd ed., pp. 116–136). Oxford University Press.

Beck, A. T. (1976). *Cognitive therapy and emotional disorders.* International Universities Press.

Beekman, L. M., Cilliers, C. D., & de Jager, A. (2012). *Student counselling and development: contemporary issues in the Southern African context.* UNISA Press.

Berg, I., & De Jong, P. (1996). Solution-building conversations: Co-constructing a sense of competence with clients. *Families in Society, 77,* 376–391.

Biglan, A., Flay, B. R., Embry, D. D., & Sandler, I. N. (2012). The critical role of nurturing environments for promoting human well-being. *American Psychologist, 67*(4), 257–271. https://doi.org/10.1037/a0026796

Bretton, M. (1993). Relating competence-promotion and empowerment. *Journal of Progressive Human Services, 5,* 27–44.

British Association for Counselling. (1989). *Invitation to membership.* B.A.C.

British Association for Counselling. (1992). *Code of ethics and practice for counsellors.* BAC.

Bruner, J. (1986). *Actual minds/possible worlds.* Harvard University.

Bruner, J. (1987). Life as narrative. *Social Research, 54,* 12–32.

Bruner, J. (1991). The narrative construction of reality. *Critical Inquiry, 18,* 1–21.

Carr, A. (1998). Michael White's narrative therapy. *Contemporary Family Therapy, 20*(4), 485–503.

Coan, G. (n.d.). *Solution-focused therapy.* Retrieved December 1, 2009, from http://ezinearticles.com/Solution-Focused-Therapy&id=10285

Corey, G. (2005). *Theory and practise of counselling and psychotherapy.* Brookes/Cole.

Crawford, T. A., & Lipsedge, M. (2004). Seeking help for psychological distress: The Interface of Zulu traditional healing and western biomedicine. *Mental Health, Religion & Culture, 7*(2), 131–148. https://doi.org/10.1080/13674670310001602463

de Shazer, S. (1985). *Keys to solution in brief therapy.* Norton.

de Shazer, S. (1994). *Words were originally magic.* Norton.

Denborough, D. (2011) Resonance, rich description and social historical healing: the use of collective narrative practice in Srebrenica. *International Journal of Narrative Therapy and Community Work, 3,* 27–42.

Dreikurs, R. (1971). *Social equality.* Alfred Adler Institute.

Dunst, C. A., Trivette, C., & Deal, A. (1988). *Enabling and empowering families.* Brookline Books.

Egan, G. (1998). *The skilled helper: A problem management approach to helping* (6th ed.). Brookes/Cole.

Evans, K., & Gilbert, M. (2009). *An introduction to integrative psychotherapy.* Palgrave Macmillan.

Gilliland, B. E., & James, R. K. (1993). Crisis intervention strategies. (2nd ed.). Brooks/Cole.

Hays, P. A. (1995). Multicultural applications of cognitive-behavior therapy. *Professional Psychology: Research and Practice, 26*, 309–315.

Knight, Z. G. (2009). Relational psychoanalysis potential usefulness with Black South African clients. *Journal of Psychology in Africa, 19*(2), 271–278.

Leahy, R. L. (2003). *Cognitive therapy techniques: A practitioner's guide.* Guilford Press.

Lee, J. A. B. (Ed.). (2001). *The empowerment approach to social work practice.* Columbia University Press.

Messer, S. B. (1992). A critical examination of belief structures in integrative and eclectic psychotherapy. In J. C. Norcross & M. R. Goldfried (Eds.), *Handbook of psychoanalytic psychotherapy.* Wiley.

Mitchell, S. A. (2000). *Relationality: From attachment to intersubjectivity.* The Analytic Press.

Mitchell, S. A., & Aron, L. (Eds.). (1999). *Relational psychoanalysis. The emergence of a tradition.* The Analytic Press.

Paul, R., & Elder, L. (2006). *The art of Socratic questioning.* Foundation for Critical Thinking.

Prilleltensky, I., & Nelson, G. (2002). *Doing psychology critically.* Pelgrave Macmillan.

Prochaska, J. O., & Norcross, J. C. (2007). *Systems of psychotherapy. A transtheoretical analysis* (6th ed.). Thomson Brooks/Cole.

Selekman, M. D. (1997). *Solution-focused therapy with children: Harnessing family strengths for systemic change.* Guilford.

Simon, B. L. (1990). Rethinking empowerment. *Journal of Progressive Human Services, 1*, 27–39.

Smith, E. J. (2006). The strength-based counseling model. *The Counseling Psychologist, 34*(1), 13–79. https://doi.org/10.1177/0011000005277018

Smith, C. (2013). Introduction. In C. Smith (Ed.), *Psychodynamic psychotherapy in contemporary South Africa: Context, theories and applications* (pp. 97–106). Wits University Press.

Smith, B. (2016). Narrative analysis. In E. Lyons & A. Coyle (Eds.). Analysing qualitative data in psychology (2nd ed) (pp. 202–221). London: Sage.

Walsh, W. B. (2004). *Counseling psychology and optimal human functioning.* Lawrence Erlbaum.

Walter, J. L., & Peller, J. E. (1992). *Becoming solution-focused in brief therapy.* Brunner/Mazel.

Wedding, D., & Corsini, R. J. (2014). *Current psychotherapies.* Brooks/Cole.

Weick, A., & Chamberlain, R. (2002). Putting problems in their place: Further explorations in the strengths perspective. In D. Saleebey (Ed.), *The strengths perspective in social work practice* (3rd ed., pp. 95–105). Allyn & Bacon.

Wolberg, L. R. (1982). *The practice of psychotherapy.* Brunner/Mazel.

Yorke, C. B., Voisin, D. R., Berringer, K. R., & Alexander, L. S. (2016). Cultural factors influencing mental health help-seeking attitudes among Black English-Speaking Caribbean immigrants in the United States and Britain. *Social Work in Mental Health, 14*(2), 174–194. https://doi.org/10.1080/15332985.2014.943832

Young, C. (2009). The transportability and utility of cognitive therapy in South African contexts: A review. *Journal of Psychology in Africa., 19*(3), 407–414.

# Chapter 8
# Contemporary Areas for Clinical Supervision Integration

Not all clients/patients may manifest pathological or clinical conditions. Some may manifest signs and symptoms of disorder, e.g. mild or moderate symptoms of anxiety or depressive disorder. Some signs and symptoms of disorder may also be triggered by situations, e.g. failure in an exam, loss of a relationship, adjustment issues or associated with certain life decisions, e.g. change of career. Unlike the pathology orientation of traditional psychotherapy, which demands historical exploration of traumas experienced in each developmental phase, the counselling context often demands a thorough contextual exploration before one can meaningfully intervene. Psychotherapists need to adopt a broad lens or advocacy approach.

## 8.1 Culture-Bound Syndrome

Another significant factor that demands a departure from traditional psychotherapy is the presentation of clients/patients with culture-bound syndromes, i.e. syndromes which are culturally unique. Swartz (2002, p. 6) views culture as 'a set of guidelines (both implicit and explicit) which individuals inherit as members of a particular society, and which tells them how to view the world, how to experience it emotionally and how to behave in relation to other people'. South Africa has a diversity of cultural groups that include African, Indian, and Islamic ideologies and practices that recognise a holistic form of psychology that includes different levels of consciousness, from subconscious to self-conscious and beyond (Assagioli, 2012; Aurobindo, 2011; Huxley, 1946; Mutwa, 2003; Wilber, 2000). In reference to these different states of consciousness, Edwards (2014) refers to ancestral consciousness which recognises departed ancestors, especially those remembered with reverence. Hinduism refers the dance of Shiva. Further, he contends that although not systemised and labelled as such, in prevalence, effect and function, such holistic, spiritual, communal psychology still remains predominant in the developing

K. V. Rawatlal, *Clinical Supervision in South Africa*, SpringerBriefs in Psychology,
https://doi.org/10.1007/978-3-031-41929-4_8

regions and countries (Edwards, 2014). This calls for an integral as well as local approach. From an integral perspective, psychology includes the study of the structures, states, modes, developmental, behavioural and relational aspects of consciousness, their manifestations in behaviour, and their application for improving humanity in particular and the universe in general (Wilber, 2000). A limited intention of this presentation is to encourage professional and student psychologists to explore their conscious and unconscious experiences towards improved insights and actions in South African and international psychological research and practice (Edwards, 2011).

In a country that includes such a diversity of ethnic groups, it is seen as unethical to continue the colonial traditions of imposing systems and ideologies of the West (Beekman et al., 2012). Naidoo (2001) proposes that psychotherapists can respond to institutional and socio-political realities through adopting an advocacy ethos, advocacy-based therapy and proactive advocacy.

In the interests of strengthening trainees' and practitioners' insight and knowledge into the different ethnic groups' ideologies, practices and worldviews, I present a brief synopsis of how illness/worldviews in the three traditions. It is important to note that the groups being referred are not homogenous and there exists various subgroupings within each of the groups. Languages may also differ in the subgroupings, the terms presented in the Islamic tradition are usually the Arabic terms, the terms in the Hindu groupings are primarily Gujarati or Hindu terms and the African tradition are primarily in the Zulu tradition (Table 8.1).

*In South Africa, **Christianity** is seen to be country's main religion, with the three top denominations being the Protestant Dutch Reformed Church, the Zion Christian Churches, and the Catholic Church. **Afrikaners** who are religious tend to be Christian, and their faith often has great prominence in their lives. Faith healers are usually professed Christians of African faith-based churches or mission-independent churches (Truter, 2007). Faith healers are called by the Holy Spirit or ancestral spirits and diagnosis and treatment is done using the Bible and praying usually using the laying of hands. Provision of holy water or ash, herbs and rituals such as animal sacrifices are often prescribed as treatment (Sodi et al., 2011).*

According to Hund (2004), the role that the healer plays is holistic as the patient seeks help for a variety of illnesses, i.e. patients may visit traditional healers for treatment of various illnesses including physical problems, divulgence of secrets, protection against witchcraft, prophecies of future events, and annual check-ups. In addition to rendering traditional medical treatments, the traditional healer also deals with 'culture-bound' syndromes that do not respond to Western treatments as with the spiritual illnesses described earlier (Hund, 2004). It is important that all health care practitioners understand the conceptualisation of spiritual illnesses and respect that whatever the practitioners' position on the existence of spiritual illnesses, for the client spiritual illness is like any other illness.

Using the Quraan and Hadith (the teachings of the Prophet Muhammed p.b.u.h) as a starting point and then the works of the early Islamic scholars, a new field has been developing in psychology termed 'Islamic Psychology'. Islamic psychology aims to promote psychological, physical and spiritual well-being. As such it is a

**Table 8.1** Synopsis of Hindu, Islamic and African Worldviews of Mental Illness and Well-being

**Hinduism** *is viewed as both a theology and a philosophy. Hindu scriptures such as the Upanishads, the Bhagavad Gita, and the Vedas; as well as the Ramayana and Mahabharata emphasise the importance of knowledge, active work, sacrifice and service to others (Chekki, 1996). Such principles are seen to provide spiritual inspiration and promote well-being. The Hindu view of mental health and illness includes magical, religious and naturalistic elements. Hinduism reflects a holistic system of beliefs which views the aspects of human nature as being independent and integrated (Fowler, 1997). Therefore, Hindu concepts of mental health cannot be separated from beliefs about physical and spiritual health. In Hinduism, there is also seen to be a thin line between mental and spiritual illness. A spiritual illness maybe construed as a mental illness and mental illness maybe misconstrued as a spiritual illness. Traditional healers in Hinduism include Gurus, Swamis, Rishis and in the management of mental illness various mantras, hymns (bhajans) and sacred phrases and words such as 'Om' and 'Shanti' are used. Amulets obtained from healers or priests are used to ward off evil. Aarti (divine light), vibbuthi (sacred ash), and natural substances like cloves, and limes are also used to treat illness (Spiro, 2005). Aarti is a Hindu religious ritual where light from wicks soaked in ghee (clarified butter) or camphor is offered to one or more deities. It is believed that the light obtains the power of the deity or deities.* **Important dates for traditional observances include Kavady and Diwali which are celebrated by Hindus worldwide.**

**The Muslim** *prayer consists of contact prayer (salaah), remembrance of Allah (zikr), and recitation of the Quraan. These forms of prayer elicit a physiologic relaxation response; prayer therefore seems to serve as a buffer against the adverse effects of stress. In the Islamic faith, traditional Healers (Moulanas, Sheikhs, or Matawaas) are the mediums through which mental illness is managed as they are considered well equipped to drive the evil spirit or the evil eye away (Sayed, 2003). Treatments for mental illness may include herbal remedies, massage therapy, Zam-Zam water (Holy water), ta'weez (amulet with Quraanic verses), water on which verses of the Quraan are read, Zam-Zam water, special Zikr and Duas (prayers). Treatment for spiritual illnesses includes ta'weez (amulet with Quraanic verses), water on which verses of the Quraan are read, ZamZam water, special Zikr and Duas, burning lobaan or other natural substances, and using herbal remedies to ease physical symptoms (Laher, 2014). Important dates for traditional observances of* **Islam include** *Eid al-Fitr and Eid al-Adha, which are* **celebrated** *by Muslims worldwide.*

*In the* **African culture**, *a Diviner in South Africa is recognised as a person who engages in traditional health practice and is registered as a diviner under the Traditional Health Practitioners Act Number 22 of 2007 (Government Gazette, 2008). The Diviner will have received a calling from the ancestors and is the most senior of healers. The Diviner protects against witchcraft and renders services to the community which include conflict resolution, revealing the cause of misfortune, recommending solutions and confirming the beliefs of patients (Sodi et al., 2011; Truter, 2007). The herbalist specialises in the use of herbal and other medicinal preparations for treating diseases and it is their individual choice to become a healer (Sodi et al., 2011). Faith healers are usually professed Christians of African faith-based churches or mission-independent churches (Truter, 2007). Faith healers are called by the Holy Spirit or ancestral spirits and diagnosis and treatment is done using the Bible and praying usually using the laying of hands. Provision of holy water or ash, herbs and rituals such as animal sacrifices are often prescribed as treatment (Sodi et al., 2011). T Treatment for illnesses in African cultures also includes cleansing measures like herbal emetics, purgatives (ukuphalaza) and enemas or laxatives (ukuchata, Edwards, 2011). These are often administered with copious amounts of fluid, sweat baths, steam baths (ukugquma), and fumigation with incense or smoke to get rid of 'polluting' or otherwise pathogenic substances (Edwards, 2011; Mpofu, 2011; Mufamadi & Sodi, 2010).*

psychology that could benefit individuals of various religions and cultures (Padayachee & Laher, 2014).

Similarly with Hinduism. Jeste and Vahia (2008), for example, cite several similarities between the Bhagavad Gita and modern scientific literature, such as rich knowledge about life, emotional regulation, insight, and a focus on common good (compassion). They argue further that the Bhagavad Gita suggests that certain components of wellness and wisdom can be taught and learned. These concepts outlined in the Gita are relevant to modern mental health in helping develop psychotherapeutic interventions that could be more holistic than those commonly practiced today as they aim at improving personal wellbeing rather than just psychiatric symptoms. Thus the use of such Hindu principles and concepts may prove beneficial in helping religious or spiritual clients, to overcome their problems in an attempt to develop a more balanced lifestyle.

African traditions also on a more holistic self in relation to the environment (Edwards, 2011; Mufamadi & Sodi, 2010). Illness is regarded as an imbalance between mind, body and spirit (Sodi et al., 2011). Spiritual illnesses form part of the categorisation of illness in African traditions (Edwards, 2011; Mpofu, 2011; Sodi et al., 2011). African traditions, like Islamic 17 and Hindu traditions, acknowledge the self as part of a larger community (see Mkhize, 2004; Mufamadi & Sodi, 2010; Sow, 1980). These commonalities between Islamic, African and Hindu understandings of self and illness are enough to argue that common ground can be found between indigenous and western approaches to health and illness that does not necessarily require the existence of separate indigenous psychologies.

It is essential that further research be done across cultures to develop a description of the symptoms and course of the three spiritual illnesses described in this paper. Collecting case studies and empirical evidence from a multitude of cultures is necessary.

## 8.2   Cultural Responsiveness Questions

In supporting trainees acquire skills to becoming culturally aware and supporting integrating indigenous knowledge in managing clients/patients' presentations, we now explore how this can be achieved. A cognitive behavioural approach, adapted from Sue et al. (2009a, b), was found to be most relevant in providing questions that provide a systematic assessment of clients/patient's subjective reality. Within this is an acknowledgement that while clients/patients may indicate they belong to a certain ethnic/religious denomination, i.e. Hinduism, Christianity, Afrocentrism, etc. not all ethnic groups are homogenous in their practice and observances of rituals and traditions.

According to Sue et al. (2009a, b) (in Sue et al., 1982, 1992) the culturally competent counsellor should have the 3 competencies given in Fig. 8.1.

Please note the questions below are not prescriptive and serve as guidelines to support health providers systematically probe into indigenous, cultural, practices,

| Cultural Awareness and Beliefs | Cultural knowledge | Cultural Skills |
|---|---|---|
| • "The provider is sensitive to her or his personal values and biases and how these may influence perceptions of the client/patient, the client's problem and the counselling relationship" (p. 4. Sue et al., 2009) | • "The health provider has knowledge of the client or patient's culture, worldview, and expectations for the counselling relationship<br>• Cultural knowledge is typically gleaned during the clinical assessment intake process, although learning about client/patient goes on throughout the treatment process<br>• It is important for the Psychologist to proactively create opportunities for clients to share their cultural perspective through asking direct and specific questions about culturally specific views. This is one way knowledge is expanded to contribute to the treatment and management plan" (p.4 Sue et al, 2009)) | • "The health provider has the ability to intervene in a manner that is culturally sensitive and relevant.<br>• Patient/Client centred skills such as empathy, non-judgemental stance, active listening skills, rapport, probing and positive regard are important to demonstrate the health providers neutral stance" (p.4. Sue et al, 2009)) |

**Fig. 8.1** Cultural competence dimensions. (Sue et al., 2009a, b)

beliefs and traditions. The health care providers' clinical judgement as to the responses elicited is important in further informing cultural tailoring of psychological intervention and management of the presenting problem (Table 8.2).

## 8.3    Telepsychology in South Africa

Another promising practice in contemporary Psychotherapy is the area of Telepsychology. There has been an evolution in the provision of Internet-based tele-communication technologies for the remote provision of psychological services (Evans, 2018). Telepsychology has thus proved popular and effective both during and in the aftermath of the COVID-19 pandemic. The potential to increase accessibility to services and reduce the stigma of seeking help has been noteworthy (Evans, 2018). Most recently, trainees have had the opportunity to experiment with

**Table 8.2** CBT + Culturally Responsive Assessment Questions for Clients/Patients

| |
|---|
| **RELIGIOUS/SPIRITUAL BELIEFS AND PRACTICES** |
| What kinds of spiritual or religious beliefs are important to you and your family? |
| Do you feel part of a religious/spiritual community? What would you like to tell me about that? |
| Do you have any favourite holidays/traditions/celebrations? Which ones are the most important for your family, and why? |
| What religious or spiritual practices do you follow? |
| Do you pray? What are your beliefs about prayer? |
| How often do you to church/temple/ashram/mosque/consult with a traditional healer/priest? |
| How do your beliefs affect your daily life? |
| **Views of mental health and mental health treatment** |
| What are your family/communities' views on counselling? |
| Does your culture have a perspective on mental health therapy or counselling? |
| Where do you or your family get help/support when a family member is experiencing a challenging time? |
| When there are troubles and needs in your family, what do you do? Who do you turn to for help? |
| What does mental health therapy or counselling mean to you? |
| Have you and anyone in your family been in counselling before? What was that like? |
| What are things your culture/tradition does that help with your sadness, anxiety, bad experiences or other troubles? |
| What were things you did in your country that helped with your sad feelings and distress? |
| Are there ways your culture has for handling trauma or other really bad life experiences? |
| **Language** |
| What languages do you speak at home vs. at school or in the community? With family vs. friends/teachers? |
| What language(s) do different family members speak at home/to each other/to others? |
| **Discrimination experiences** |
| Have you ever been treated poorly because of your beliefs/ethnicity/race, etc.? What are some of the ways you have been treated poorly? |
| Have you ever felt different from others because of your beliefs/ethnicity/race, etc. What are some of the ways you felt different? |
| What are some of the wrong assumptions people have made about you and your family that have caused problems? |
| **General/nonspecific concluding questions** |
| I have asked you a lot of questions. Do you have any questions for me about the assessment/counselling? Is there something you want to tell me that we haven't talked about? |
| What are some of the things I may have missed in the questions I've asked? |
| Do you go by any other name than what is indicated? What name would you like me to call you? |
| Is there anything else about your background, culture or identity that you think is important for me to know to help you? |

Adapted from Sue et al. (2009a, b)

the platform in their practicum training at Student Counselling sites and primary health care facilities. It has been pleasing to note that an increase in clients/patients has emanated from such practices and trainees have also provided positive feedback of how this has contributed to strengthening their therapeutic skills.

In Telepsychology, different technologies maybe used in various combinations and for different purposes in the provision of telepsychology services (Evans, 2018).

Services maybe provided via email, text messaging, video conferencing, websites, chatrooms or forums. The communication can also be synchronous where parties communicate in real time (e.g. email) or even non-interactional (e.g. psychoeducational websites). Telepsychology can be used as an adjunct to traditional face-to-face services or it can be used on its own.

Evans (2018) discusses guidelines for the practice of Telepsychology in South Africa and refers to the need for the provision of such guidelines to promote ethical standards for psychology given the fast-changing nature of technology and the potential impact on the field. It is also advised that practitioners consult with the Revised General Ethical Guidelines for Good Practice in Telemedicine Registered with the Health Professions Council of South Africa (HPCSA, 2020), Booklet 10 to further guide their practice. Trainee practitioners should also adhere to the memorandum of agreement at their respective sites regarding the telepsychology consultations. All trainee Psychologists should be registered as Student Psychologists with the Health Professions Council of South Africa before they commence their practicum work. Table 8.3. represents some of the key areas trainees need to consider in facilitating telepsychology consultation sessions in their practicum work. For more in-depth information, the author refers to Evans (2018), *Some guidelines for telepsychology in South Africa* and the HPCSA (2020) *Revised General Ethical Guidelines for Good Practice in Telemedicine.* Some practical considerations are also discussed.

### 8.3.1   Some Practical Considerations

The American Psychological Association (APA, 2013) defines 'telepsychology' as 'the provision of psychological services using telecommunication technologies' (p. 3). Telepsychology includes several methods of therapeutic services, such as videoconferencing, instant messaging and online chat (McCord et al., 2021). Guidelines for practicing teletherapy include competency of the technology and therapeutic services to ensure that ethical and professional standards of care are met (APA, 2013). It is important to obtain informed consent that specifically addresses concerns with telepsychology services. Also, it is important to ensure confidentiality and privacy with the increased risks inherent to the use of telecommunication technologies.

## 8.4   How to Set Up the Session

It is essential to ensure proper setup for teletherapy sessions. This section will go over considerations of what to do before, during, and after the session. The following considerations are adapted from APA (2013) and Galpin et al. (2020).

**Table 8.3**  Adapted Guidelines for Telepsychology from Evans (2018)

**1. Best interests of the client/patients**

Psychologists should always use their clinical judgement to consider if telepsychology is an appropriate service for the client and not only the most feasible option.

Psychologists should continually assess whether telepsychology is an appropriate service to meet the client/patients presenting needs and, if it is not, then refer clients to alternative in-person services. In all instances, it is extremely important that the trainee be totally present. Telepsychology may be contraindicated if the:

Client/patient has a high-risk status in terms of suicidality and/or homicidality.

Client/patient's current **global assessment of functioning** (GAF) is low.

Client/patient is not competent in using, or does not have access to, the technology required.

**2. Competence**

Evans (2018) refers to as part of a psychologist's competence they should be able to provide telepsychology within the boundaries of their professional competence derived from their training, registration and professional experience. Further, he indicates the need for Psychologists to engage in ongoing professional development in telepsychology to maintain their competence. Competence also refers to the Psychologist being competent in using the technology required to perform telepsychology and having the skills to manage any potential risks posed by the technology. Lastly, he refers to Psychologists ensuring that clients are competent in using the technology and that they may need to assist clients to gain the necessary skills.

**3. Confidentiality**

In engaging clients/patients on this platform, psychologists should take all reasonable, precautionary efforts to protect and maintain the confidentiality of data/information. The institution or practicum site you may find yourself will require all clients to sign an informed consent form that indicates the agreement between the client and the psychologist. This consent form also protects the confidentiality of information shared. The patient must at all times be assured that their confidentiality is protected. Patient confidentiality should be ensured at both the consulting and servicing practitioners' sites and should follow the provisions of the Constitution, the National Health Act No 61 of 2003, the Promotion of Access to Information Act No 2 of 2000, the Protection of Personal Information Act No 4 of 2013, the Common law and the HPCSA's ethical guidelines on patient confidentiality in Booklet 10 which generally state that it is every practitioner's duty to make sure that information is effectively protected against improper disclosure at all times.

According to Evan's (2018) precautionary efforts should also include: Protecting devices (especially mobile devices) with a secure password to prevent unauthorised access; installation and updating of antivirus software; password protecting any confidential documents sent via email or any other communication medium; ensuring that any communication does not reach unintended recipients; ensuring that a secure platform is used to data storage of a client's records; ensuring that when data and/or devices need to be disposed that no third party can access or recover the confidential data; ensuring that both the psychologist and client use a private, confidential environment when engaging in telepsychology.

**4. Professional boundaries**

In telepsychology, it is important for trainees to maintain appropriate professional boundaries and at the same level of professionalism regardless of the communication used. This means that they should communicate the limits to their availability (i.e. working hours); negotiate the purposes that different communication mediums can be used for (e.g. email for administrative purposes and video-conferencing for therapeutic purposes), clarify the anticipated response times when using asynchronous communication mediums and avoid 'befriending' clients on social media platforms. Psychologists should also respect a client's privacy and refrain from doing internet searches to find out about a client, unless the client has consented.

(continued)

**Table 8.3**  (continued)

| |
|---|
| **5. Crisis management** |
| Trainees may sometimes also experience different emergency situations (e.g. suicidality, self-mutilation) when using telepsychology, as clients/patients are often not in the same location as the psychologist providing the service. Evans (2018) indicates that Psychologists should therefore prepare for future emergency situations by:<br>    Developing a crisis support plan collaboratively with their client<br>    Obtaining the contact details of the client's next of kin or another preferred personal emergency contact<br>    Determining, in collaboration with the client, local supports and local health-care providers that can be used in emergency situations<br>    Establishing which methods should be used in an emergency situation to ensure their availability. |

- Consultation room set up

  - The virtual and physical space should be professional, confidential and free from distractions.
  - The practitioner should ideally position themselves with a wall in the background so that there is no potential for people distracting or viewing the session.
  - Practitioners should consider having minimal personal items and distracting patterns in the background.
  - The room should be well lit and the camera angle should be appropriate to ensure the client can see you.

- Technology set up

  - Make sure that the internet connectivity is secure and adequate. The practitioner also advises the client to confirm that the settings are adequate on their end.
  - The picture and audio quality should also be checked to ensure that the client can clearly see and hear the practitioner.

- Session set up

  - Confirm the client's location beforehand and identify emergency resources such as the nearest hospital or emergency number, in case any medical or mental health emergency arises. Confirm also alternative communication channels if the client loses connectivity.
  - Ensure the client is in a state in which you are able to provide services. If they are not, teletherapy may not be appropriate.

- Provide resources to clients

  - Provide the client with information on how to log in and use the technology needed for telehealth services.
  - Be able to explain to clients what makes the platform secure, and how users can inadvertently limit privacy and confidentiality. Some sites may have an informed consent form for teletherapy which the practitioner may need to discuss with the client.
  - Discussing case management with the client before the start of any clinical service is helpful.

## 8.5   Telehealth Microskills

Clinical microskills are fundamental in providing therapeutic services. However, it is even more imperative in providing teletherapy. When providing teletherapy some skills may need to be modified to ensure they are not being lost in translation or misinterpreted. The following is from Galpin et al. (2020), McCord et al. (2021) and Myers and Turvey (2013).

## 8.6   Body Language and Voice

In face-to-face clinical work, clinicians attempt to convey empathy and connection through use of eye contact, body positioning and facial expressions. These may become lost and not translate well through an online platform. Here are some tips to alter them and convey that same warmth you want:

### 8.6.1   Eye Contact

Make sure that you are looking at the camera of your computer to convey eye contact. Another tip can be to sit slightly further away from your camera than normal so that there is more 'room' for your gaze to move without it appearing as breaking eye contact.

### 8.6.2   Body Positioning

Make sure you take up the majority of space in your video box, and show the upper part of your body. You may need to adjust the camera so that it cuts off the very top of your hairline or head so that clients can see your torso. This can also help with modelling for the clients how you would like them to set up their own camera and video themselves.

### 8.6.3   Facial Expressions

Practitioners need to be present and genuinely interested in what their clients are saying and try to mirror their reactions. Because you will see yourself as well, consider covering that box up if it is distracting to you. You should adjust the lighting in the room to avoid unsightly shadows or backlighting on your face. Appropriate lighting of your face will allow for your facial expressions to be clearly seen.

### 8.6.4   Tone

Make sure to have a warm tone of voice similar to what you may use in an in-person session. It is easy for us to sometimes speak louder when on tele-platforms, so be sure to modulate your voice. Check the quality of your microphone. If the microphone causes your voice to come across as muffled or unclear, the tone of your voice will not be heard.

## 8.7   Flexibility and Establishing Rapport

- Technology issues can arise at any time, so be sure that there are multiple options for communication, in case one fails.
    - For example, if video calling is not possible, do you have the capabilities to switch to a phone call?
- Establishing rapport includes reassuring that teletherapy is a valid and reliable service delivery model. Reiterating the purpose of telehealth delivery can help ease the client's concerns.
- Clinicians can also establish rapport by responding to any changes to the client's body language and emotions, and offering them choices when appropriate.

### 8.7.1   Managing Technological Issues

Having a reliable technological system for providing teletherapy services is of great importance. However, technical issues may arise and it is critical to be prepared for them. The following points are from McCord et al. (2021):

Preparing for a technological issue:

- At the onset of services, it is important to communicate plans if there are outages or downtime in the telepsychology services.
    - For example, if the videoconferencing system is unstable a plan can be set for the clinician to contact the client by phone. Once contacted by phone the clinician and client can discuss options on how to continue. If possible, offer to continue services over the phone.
- It is important to explain to the client that technological issues are infrequent but an aspect of teletherapy.
- Maintaining clear and consistent communication is important through technical difficulties so the client does not feel unsure and abandoned.

## 8.8   Record Keeping

- It is important to maintain notes of all contacts with the client.
- It is important to distinguish the type of service modality that has been used.

  – For example, was the modality of services in-person, videoconferencing, or telephone.

- It is important to note the duration of the phone contact or teletherapy session.

  – For example, the phone contact lasted 5 mins, the therapy session was a total of 52 minutes (42 minutes with the adolescent and 10 minutes with the father).

- It is important to note the location of the client in the documentation when providing telepsychological services.

  – For example, the counsellor can ask at the beginning of the session for the address of their location.

- It is important to keep all notes and forms private and secure when conducting telepsychological services.

  – For example, make sure you are maintaining documentation on the secure platform as directed by the training clinic. Do not maintain or keep documentation on your personal platforms.

### 8.8.1   Diversity Considerations

Diversity and multicultural components should always be recognised when providing therapeutic and teletherapy services. Teletherapy possesses multicultural considerations that are built upon foundational multicultural counselling considerations. All diversity and multicultural components of teletherapy need to be acknowledged and addressed. These considerations are adapted from APA (2013), APA (2017), Galpin et al. (2020) and McCord et al. (2021).

Considerations include:

### 8.8.2   Socio-economic Barriers

- Socio-economic gaps in access to technology may impair clients' technology literacy. For example, clients who do not have access to a personal computer may feel uncomfortable receiving teletherapy. Also, older clients who are not experienced in using technology may not feel comfortable with teletherapy.

- The client's socioeconomic status may prohibit access to services. For example, if the client does not have access to a computer, stable form of internet, and a secure and private location they may not be able to receive teletherapy services.
- Socio-economic status is also often intertwined with race and ethnicity, so in addition to SES, clinicians can also consider how these accessibility issues relate to race and ethnicity.

### 8.8.3 Nonverbal Barriers

- Nonverbal cultural data is unavailable. Full-body language and gestures are not seen on telehealth platforms. For example, depending on the client's culture their eye contact can vary. On telehealth platforms, it may be very difficult to identify this.

### 8.8.4 Clinician Evaluation

- It is important for a clinician to evaluate and address personal biases.
- It is important for a clinician to develop cultural awareness. The clinician's cultural awareness should include how clinicians view culture in the context of the client conceptualisation, diagnosis, treatment plan, and interventions.
- It is important for a clinician to be open to talking about culture throughout the therapeutic process. This models to the client that these conversations are welcomed and warranted in the assessment.

## 8.9 Phototherapy

The postmodern and social constructivist era in Psychology presents an opportunity for Psychologists to utilise creative and therapeutic techniques that will offer the most support for the client/patient's individual needs. One art therapy technique that has been utilised in mainstream counselling and psychotherapy is Phototherapy. Phototherapy involves taking, viewing, manipulating and interpreting photographs as a primary or adjunct therapeutic technique (Hayes, 2002; Krauss & Fryrear, 1983).

Having a concrete image to make reference to allows both the client and therapist to share an understanding (Buchalter, 2009; McNiff, 2004). The therapist is able to provide an objective viewpoint and feedback that the client might not have considered otherwise. The utilisation of images in therapy allows the clients to externalise their difficulties, situations, feelings and discuss them in therapy in a more objective manner (Ginicola et al., 2012). Schudson (1975) also indicates that phototherapy can help the counsellor and client in all stages of counselling that include building

**Table 8.4** Phototherapy intervention strategies

| Strategies | References |
|---|---|
| ***Self-portraits, telling narratives through pictures, exploring symbols/objects***<br>In terms of treatment strategies, research indicates that explorations of **self and self-confrontation** can be employed through self-portraits, telling narratives through pictures and explorations of self through symbols. | Glover-Graf and Miller (2006), Hunsberger (1984), Pillay (2009), Reynolds et al. (2008) and Star and Cox (2008) |
| ***Exploring positive and negative relationships***<br>Photography has also been used to understand and explore both positive and negative relationships. | Goessling and Doyle (2009), Hays et al. (2009), Krauss and Fryrear (1983), Loewenthal (2009a, b), Reynolds et al. (2008), Star and Cox (2008), Weiser (2004a, b) and Wessells (1985) |
| ***Analysis of dreams and experiences***<br>Photographs have been used to help the client examine and analyse memories and experiences | Goodhart et al. (2006), Hanieh and Walker (2007), Krauss and Fryrear (1983), Schudson (1975) and Star and Cox (2008) |
| ***Coping skills and solutions***<br>The photographs also help to explore alternative behavioural responses by exploring coping skills and solutions | Rhodes and Hergenrather (2007) |
| ***Process of change towards termination of psychotherapy***<br>Phototherapy can also assist with proper termination with the client. Previous research shows that investigating the development of the photos through the counselling sessions can indicate and document the process of change. Phototherapy has also been significantly associated with feelings of empowerment, achievement and creativity, which will help the client leave with positive feelings, concrete copings skills and a visual representation of their time in therapy | Krauss and Fryrear (1983), Goessling and Doyle (2009), Goodhart et al. (2006), Krauss and Fryrear (1983) and Reynolds et al. (2008) |

rapport and trust. The intervention has been evidenced to serve as an alternative form of communication and found to lower anxiety surrounding communication through eliciting higher rates of verbal communication Goodhart et al., 2006; Krauss & Fryrear, 1983; Reynolds et al., 2008; Schudosn, 1975). Also significantly, in reference to indigenous knowledge practices and traditions, discussed earlier, the counsellor can also explore the client's cultural influences, meanings and spirituality by reviewing the content and discussing its importance for the client (Goessling & Doyle, 2009; Hays et al., 2009; Loewenthal, 2009a, b; Reynolds et al., 2008). Some specific treatment strategies that Phototherapy intervention enables are now discussed (Table 8.4).

In considering the clinical use of photography, the application of photographs in clinical and therapeutic contexts has grown significantly in recent years (Loewenthal, 2013). Empirical evidence confirms how images can activate and facilitate the communication of thoughts and emotions without the limitations of verbal language, which then contributes to overcome challenges of difficulties some individuals may experience (Uhrig et al., 2016). As trainees are confronted with working with vulnerable clients/patient populations, whose presentations and the management thereof, are sometimes hindered by limitations of verbal language, the use of phototherapy is seen to have potential. It must however be noted that Phototherapy should not be used exclusively but rather as an intervention to supplement or support other theory-based psychotherapeutic interventions. This in reference to a systemic review of the literature conducted by Saita and Tramontano (2018) which concluded that 'despite its increasing use as an intervention methodology, not many scientific papers concerning the clinical and therapeutic use of photography are currently present in the literature' (pg. 10, Saita & Tramontano, 2018).

## 8.10   Career Counsellor Competencies for the Twenty-First Century

Kim et al. (2002) describe career counselling as similar in nature to traditional counselling. Many aspects and skills of personal counselling are seen as essential in career counselling (Sharf, 2006) and most significantly, a concern with the whole person as they seek to come to an understanding of themselves, their aims and values (Malan, 1999). In practice, a career problem is often only the beginning point whereafter other problems emerge. Career issues often become personal-emotional and family issues and then career issues again (Gysbers et al., 2003). Schultheiss (2000, p. 43) proposes an integrated view of personal and career issues.

Competencies Psychologists should have to facilitate career transitions include the following below, adapted from Beekman et al. (2012) (Table 8.5).

Navigating 'All or nothing' thinking in career counselling.

In this postmodern era, it is seen as most significant for Psychologists to support clients to reflect on a 'career cycle' as a cycle that both challenges and reinforces many of the traditional irrational messages regarding careers (Richman, 1988). The myth that in order to achieve success, clients must follow a straight and narrow path throughout their career cycle, may lead clients avoidance in defining career goals. When the career cycle is viewed in 'all-or-nothing terms', without considering other

**Table 8.5**  An integrated view of personal and career issues

| |
|---|
| Specific knowledge and skills on a scholarship level (that includes career and guidance theory knowledge in order to practice from a theory-driven conceptual framework |
| Trends and labour market knowledge in order to interpret changes in the career landscape and translate it to students and stakeholders to facilitate facts-based decision making |
| Knowledge about different career fields, study programmes (both national and international) vocations, job profiles and requirements |
| Knowledge about resources for career development such as placement agencies, vacation work, learnerships and employment opportunities |
| Knowledge of assessment instruments and the skill to use different methods and techniques to facilitate exploration, career planning and life design |

options, or that each stage must be completed within an exact age range and in one set direction, the entire concept of career may serve as a deterrent for many clients and increase their fear of pursuing satisfying career goals. Modifying internal beliefs which interfere with achieving career goals at all stages of the career cycle is therefore seen as an essential part of the process.

Career counsellors will be required to integrate career and mental health counselling interventions in their work with clients impacted by the COVID-19 pandemic. Specifically, there will likely be an increased need for career development professionals who are proficient in trauma-informed care. Trauma-informed career counselling approaches include (a) establishing an environment of trust and safety, (b) assessing for trauma-related symptoms, (c) use of ecological frameworks to conceptualise associations between traumatic experiences and work, (d) developing healthy coping strategies and (e) promoting career adaptability (Barrow et al., 2019). Career counselling interventions should also focus on basic survival, social, and self-determination needs that have been eroded by pandemic-related precarious work or underemployment, as these all relate to psychological well-being (Duffy et al., 2016). For example, helping clients identify avenues outside of work to fulfil social connection needs may be necessary to mitigate the effects of social isolation caused by remote work (Duffy et al., 2016). Supporting clients to assess their personal strengths and prior acts of resilience may aid in developing coping strategies for current work-related stressors and foster a renewed sense of self-determination. Lastly, supporting clients broaden their social support networks may supplement their survival needs that have been jeopardised by turbulent economic times.

### 8.10.1  Approaching from a Cognitive Behavioural Perspective

Beyond supporting clients develop skills, as referred to in the previous paragraph, in applying an action theoretical perspective (Chen, 1999; Collin & Young, 1986) highlight how career counsellors can help clients frame their career exploration and planning in a joint-action context. The conceptualisation of joint action can actually be illustrated and naturally integrated through the entire counselling process. In revisiting past experiences, a client may become realise that significant others, for example, family members and friends, were co-participants in his/her action (Chen, 1999; Collin & Young, 1986).

Also, in drawing attention to immediacy, the client recognises that the ongoing client-counsellor working alliance is a demonstration of joint action. Further, in projecting future career, the client is encouraged to have consultation with family members and/or trusted ones in life, representing a joint action effort. Most significantly, individual action or agency is well situated in a joint action context. Career counselling can thus facilitate the joint action-oriented agentic implementation, addressing and reflecting a variety of complex social dimensions in the client's personal and vocational life pursuits. Strengthening and implementing a sense of joint action appears to be consistent in promoting clients' agentic function within the macro-ecology of life career development (Chen, 1999; Collin & Young, 1986).

Integrating action and agency in persons' life career development is best actualised in contextual narratives (Cochran, 1997; Young & Valach, 1996). Human beings are seen to live narrative lives. Every moment of being follows the narrative flow that comprises cognitive, affective, and behavioural experiences (Polkinghorne, 1988; Sarbin, 1986). Personal life and worklife integrate in a natural way, and they are constructed and progress with rich meanings enclosed (Peavy, 1993; Savickas, 1991). Career pathing is seen to represent a narrative construction that conveys text content, plots, and climax to organise critical meanings in human action and experiences.

The narrative approach is particularly relevant in facilitating a meaning making and meaning-interpretation process, which pinpoints the very essence of career counselling, that is, understand the meaning of career, or in Cochran's (1990) term, a sense of vocation. The counselling process keeps the goal of facilitating clients' positive change and growth through their own narration so that a victim's and patient's script would be transformed into the story of an agent and actor who makes things happen (Cochran, 1997).

Meanwhile, counselling must keep in mind and address the complexity and multiplicity of human action as proposed by action theory, aiming to promote and facilitate a more holistic approach in projecting and implementing project in people's worklife and vocational development (Young, 2001).

In career counselling practice, making clients unlearn mindset (core beliefs and all or nothing thinking) or asking them to see a perspective completely foreign to them is challenging to them. Misinformed foundational/core beliefs about self-concept, stigma, prejudice, gender bias are prevalent in client's presentations for career counselling. The pressure of being selected into highly competitive programmes that only select few candidates. Such programmes are also based on equity and employment goals which force ideally suited clients to compromise and consider second and third career options. This mindset needs to be confronted and requires patience and persistence from the Psychologist. Encouraging a sense of agency and motivation is seen as key and challenging patterns of behaviour and 'all or nothing' thinking can take a lot longer than anticipated in making a decision. From this mindset, addressing the cognitive barriers which hinder successful career development is pivotal.

## 8.10.2   Strengths-Based Case Management and Conceptualisation

In reference to contextual factors that influence therapeutic outcomes, the strengths-based model of case management is seen as most relevant. The model is based on the theory of strengths and aims to identify factors that are impacting an individual's

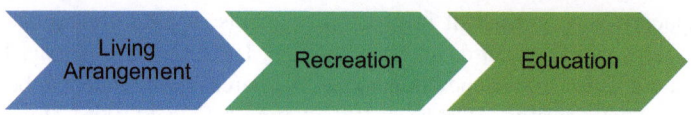

**Fig. 8.2  Domains that impact client's lives**

life and how they can be changed (Arnold et al., 2007). The theory highlights that clients must identify their own desired outcomes in areas such as the quality of their life, achievement, sense of competency, life satisfaction and empowerment. The theory identifies the different domains that clients live in (Arnold et al., 2007) and are considered important for practitioners to assess. The listed points in Fig. 8.2 are seen to directly impact the achievement of these outcomes.

In turn, individual factors such as *aspirations, competencies, confidence and environmental* (e.g. resources, social relations, opportunities, strengths) directly impact the quality of these individual domains. The theory is based on internal as well as external factors that impact clients' lives.

**The Strengths-based case management model (SBCM) in based on six principles (C.A. Rapp,** 1998) **(Table 8.6).**

Core to the SBCM is the practitioner's engagement and the development of a relationship with clients, strengths assessment, personal planning, resource acquisition and ongoing collaboration and gradual disengagement (Rapp, 1998).

Over time, the more general DSM system has come under critical review, especially by counsellors who question how the diagnostic process fits with professional identity and ethical obligation (Eriksen & Kress; Kress et al., 2010; Zalaquett et al., 2008). Limitations of the DSM require that counsellors use it carefully, and thoughtfully consider challenges related to its use. Eriksen and Kress (2005) wrote in reference to the most recent DSM-IV-TR, underlying assumptions and broad-based diagnostic processes as not having changes in the DSM-5 (APA, 2013). Kress et al. (2010) indicate that the limitations of this diagnostic and classification system will continue to be relevant.

Before the limitations are discussed, the literature identifies that the DSM system is useful in a number of ways (APA, 2013; Dailey et al., 2014; Eriksen & Kress, 2005, 2006; Kress & Paylo, 2014). Primarily, it serves as a way of communicating about client problems and struggles. Assuming that all client-related information is considered, it offers a vehicle for reducing complex information into a manageable form (Kress & Paylo, 2014). Through the categorisation of psychological symptoms into disorders, the DSM classification system provides a means for counsellors to select evidence-based treatments that correspond to the said disorder. According to Kress and Paylo (2014) some clients may benefit from receiving a diagnosis as it may help them to normalise and understand their experiences, sometimes even helping them to reduce the shame and self-blame often related to symptoms (Eriksen & Kress, 2005).

**Table 8.6** Strengths-based case management model

| |
|---|
| 1. The focus is on an individual strength rather than pathology |
| 2. The community is viewed as an oasis of resources |
| 3. Interventions are based on client self-determination |
| 4. The case manager-client relationship is primary and essential |
| 5. Aggressive outreach is the preferred mode of intervention |
| 6. People can learn, grow and change |

Categorisation (mild, moderate, severe) and identification of mental disorders supports counsellors/clinicians with prevention, early intervention and effective treatment and management plans.

**It is important for trainees to be mindful that reporting a *DSM* diagnosis is only one part of a comprehensive assessment**. What one reports in terms of diagnosis is just a 'snapshot' of the client. A comprehensive assessment needs to capture both the strengths and areas for development of the client/patient. Any comprehensive assessment must take into account an understanding of all relevant factors. These would also include, but are not only limited to, psychosocial factors such as psychological symptoms, family interactions, developmental factors, contextual factors, functional abilities longitudinal-historical information. Communication of diagnosis information is seen to play a critical role in adherence to the treatment and management plan and in some cases, the prevention of the manifestation of severe forms of pathology. Along with a humanistic, strength- and competency-based perspective, practitioners need to also be sensitive to contextual and cultural considerations. Reference is made to the DSM-IV Axis V Codes. Axis V refers to Psychosocial and Environmental factors Whereby clinicians can simply note salient environmental factors (Probst, 2014, p. 123). This would include notation regarding concerns in 9 key areas that include primary support group, social environment, education, occupation, housing, economy, access to health care; legal system/crime, and others (APA, 2000).

# References

American Psychiatric Association (2000). Diagnostic and statistical manual of mental disorders (4th ed. text rev.) Washinton DC: Author.

American Psychological Association. (2017). *Ethical principles of psychologists and code of conduct*. Retrieved from https://www.apa.org/ethics/code

American Psychiatric Association. (2013). *Diagnostic and statistical manual of mental disorders* (5th ed.). Author.

Arnold, E. M., Walsh, A. K., Oldham, M. S., & Rapp, C. A. (2007). Strengths based case management: Implementation with high risk youth. Families in Society: The Journal of Contemporary Social Services. https://doi.org/10.1606/1044-3894.3595

Assagioli, R. (2012). *Psychosynthesis. A collection of basic writing*. The Synthesis Centre.

Aurobindo, S. (2011). *The integral yoga*. Lotus Press.

Barrow, J., Wasik, S. Z., Corry, L. B., & Gobble, C. A. (2019). Trauma-informed career counseling: Identifying and advocating for the vocational needs of human services clients and professionals. *Journal of Human Services, 39*, 97–110.

Beekman, L., Cilliers, S., & De Jager, A. (2012). *Student counselling and developing. Contemporary issues in the Southern African context.* UNISA Press, South Africa.

Buchalter, S. I. (2009). *Art therapy techniques and applications: A model for practice.* Jessica Kingsley.

Chen, C. P. (1999). Human agency in context. Toward an ecological frame of career counselling. *Guidance and Counselling, 14*(3), 3–10.

Chekki, D. A. (1996). Family values and family change. *Journal of Comparative Family Studies, 27*(2), 409–413.

Cochran, L. (1990). *The sense of vocation: A study of career and life development.* State University of New York Press.

Cochran, L. (1997). *Career counseling: A narrative approach.* Sage.

Collin, A., & Young, R. A. (1986). New directions for theories of career. *Human Relations, 39*(9), 837–853.

Dailey, S. F., Gill, C. S., Karl, S. L., & Barrio Minton, C. A. (2014). *DSM-5 learning companion: A guide for counselors.* American Counseling Association.

Duffy, R. D., Blustein, D. L., Diemer, M. A., & Autin, K. L. (2016). The psychology of working theory. *Journal of Counseling Psychology, 63*(2), 127–148. https://doi.org/10.1037/cou0000140

Edwards, S. D. (2011). A psychology of indigenous healing in South Africa. *Journal of Psychology in Africa, 21*, 335–348.

Edwards, S. D. (2014). Integral approach to South African psychology with special reference to indigenous knowledge. *Journal of Psychology in Africa, 24*(6), 526–532.

Eriksen, K., & Kress, V. E. (2005). *Beyond the DSM story: Ethical quandaries, challenges, and best practices.* Sage.

Eriksen, K., & Kress, V. E. (2006). The DSM and professional counseling identity: Bridging the gap. *Journal of Mental Health Counseling, 28*, 202–217.

Evans, D. J. (2018). Some guidelines for telepsychology in South Africa. *South Africa Journal of Psychology, 48*(2), 166–170.

Fowler, J. (1997). *Hinduism: Beliefs and practices.* Sussex Academic Press.

Galpin, K., Sikka, N., King, S. L., Horvath, K. A., Shipman, S. A., Telehealth Advisory, A. A. M. C., & Committee. (2020). Expert consensus: Telehealth skills for health care professionals. *Telemedicine and e-Health, 27*(7), 820–824.

Ginicola, M. M., Smith, C., & Trzaska, J. (2012). Using photography in counselling: Images of healing. *The International Journal of the Image, 2*(2), 29–24.

Glover-Graf N. M., Miller E. (2006). The use of phototherapy in group treatment for persons who are chemically dependent. *Rehabilitation Counseling Bulletin, 49*, 166–181. https://doi.org/10.1177/00343552060490030401

Goodhart, F., Hsu, J., Baek, J. H., Coleman, A. L., Maresca, F. M., & Miller, M. B. (2006). View through a different lens: Photovoice as a tool for student advocacy. *Journal of American College Health, 55*(1), 53–56. https://doi.org/10.3200/JACH.55.1.53-56

Goessling, K., & Doyle, C. (2009). Thru the Lenz: Participatory action research, photography, and creative process in an urban high school. *Journal of Creativity in Mental Health, 4*(4), 343–365. https://doi.org/10.1080/15401380903375979

Government Gazette. (2008). Traditional Health Practitioners Act 22 of 2007. http://www.polity.org.za/article/traditional-health-practitioners-act-no-22-of-2007-2008-01-31

Gysbers, N. C., Heppner, M. J., & Johnson, J. A. (2003). *Career counselling: Process, issues and techniques* (2nd ed.). Allyn & Bacon.

Hanieh, E., & Walker B. M. (2007). Photography as a measure of constricted construing the experience of depression through a camera. *Journal of Constructivist Psychology, 20*, 183–200. https://doi.org/10.1080/10720530601074739

Hayes, D. (2002). Photography: Snapshots out of the unconscious. *Psychodynamic Practice: Individuals, Groups and Organisations, 8*(4), 525–532. https://doi.org/10.1080/1353333021000038863

Hays, D. G., Forman, J., & Sikes, A. (2009). Using artwork and photography to explore adolescent females' perceptions of dating relationships. *Journal of Creativity in Mental Health, 4*(4), 295–307. https://doi.org/10.1080/15401380903385960

Health Professions Council of South Africa. (2020). *Guidance on the application of telemedicine guidelines during the COVID-19 pandemic.* HPCSA. https://www.hpcsa.co.za/Uploads/Events/Announcements/APPLICATION_OF_TELEMEDICINE_GUIDELINES.pdf. Accessed 12 Apr 2020

Hund, J. (2004). African Witchcraft and Western law: Psychological and cultural issues. *Journal of Contemporary Religion, 19*, 67–84.

Hunsberger, P. (1984). Uses of instant-print photography in psychotherapy. Professional Psychology: *Research and Practice, 15*(6), 884–890. https://doi.org/10.1037/0735-7028.15.6.884

Huxley, A. (1946). *The perennial philosophy.* Fontana.

Jeste, D. V., & Vahia, I. V. (2008). Comparison of the conceptualization of wisdom in ancient Indian literature with modern views: Focus on the Bhagavad Gita. *Psychiatry, 71*, 197–209.

Kim, B. S., Li, L. C., & Lian, C. T. (2002). Effects of Asian American client adherence to Asian cultural values, session goal, and counsellor emphasis of client expression on career counselling process. *Journal of Counselling Psychology, 49*(3), 342–354.

Krauss, D. A., & Fryrear, J. (1983). *Phototherapy in mental health.* Charles C. Thomas.

Kress, V. E., Hoffman, R. M., & Eriksen, K. (2010). Ethical dimensions of diagnosing: Considerations for clinical mental health counselors. *Counseling and Values, 55*, 101–112. https://doi.org/10.1002/j.2161-007X.2010.tb00024.x

Kress, V. E., & Paylo, M. J. (2014). *Treating those with mental disorders: A comprehensive approach to case conceptualization and treatment.* Pearson.

Laher, S. (2014). An overview of illness conceptualizations in African, Hindu, and Islamic traditions: Towards cultural competence. *South Africa Journal of Psychology, 44*, 191–204. https://doi.org/10.1177/0081246314528149

Loewenthal, D. (2009a). Can photographs help one ind one's voice? The use of photographs in the psychological therapies. *European Journal of Psychotherapy and Counselling, 11*(1), 1–6. https://doi.org/10.1080/13642530902745804

Loewenthal, D. (2009b). Editorial. European Journal of Psychotherapy and Therapeutic Photography in a digital age. In D. Loewenthal (Ed.), *Phototherapy and therapeutic photographs in a digital age* (pp. 5–20). Routledge.

Loewenthal, D. (2013). *Photherapy and Therapeutic Photography in a Digital Age.* Routledge. London.

Malan, F. (1999). *Facing the future.* Collegium.

McNiff, S. (2004). *Art heals: How creativity cures the soul.* Random House.

Mutwa, V. C. (2003). *Zulu shaman. Dreams, prophecies and mysteries.* Destiny Books.

McCord, C. E., Console, K., Jackson, K., Palmiere, D. M., Stickley, D. M., Williamson, M. L. C., & Armstrong, T. W. (2021). Telepsychology training in a public health crisis: A case example. *Counselling Psychology Quarterly, 34*(3–4), 608–623. https://doi.org/10.1080/09515070.2020.1782842

Mkhize, N. (2004). Psychology: An African perspective. In D. Hook (Ed.), *Critical psychology* (pp. 24–52). UCT Press.

Mpofu, E. (2011). Counselling people of African ancestry. Cambridge University Press

Mufamadi, J., & Sodi, T. (2010). Notions of mental illness by Vhavenda traditional healers in Limpopo Province, South Africa. *Indilinga African Journal of Indigenous Knowledge Systems, 9*, 253–264. Elsevier.

Myers, K., & Turvey, C. L. (2013). *Telemental health: Clinical, technical, and administrative foundations for evidence-based practice.* Waltham.

Naidoo, L.R. (2001). Advocacy: Student counselling's response to the social healing curriculum. Paper presented at the National Conference of the Society for Student Counselling in Souther Africa. Cape Technikon, Cape Town.

Padayachee, P., & Laher, S. (2014). Hindu psychologists perceptions of mental illness. *Journal of Religion and Health, 53*, 424–443.

Peavy, R. V. (1993). Envisioning the future: Worklife and counselling. *Canadian Journal of Counselling, 27*, 123–139.

Pillay, Y. (2009). The use of digital narratives to enhance counselingand psychotherapy. *Journal of Creativity in Mental Health, 4*(1), 32–41. https://doi.org/10.1080/15401380802705375

Polkinghorne, D. E. (1988). *Narrative knowing and the human sciences.* State University of New York Press.

Probst, B. (2014). The life and death of sxis IV: Caught in the quest for a theory of mental disorder. *Research on Social Work Practice, 24*, 123–131.

Reynolds, F., Lim, K., & Prior, S. (2008). Images of resistance: A qualitative enquiry into the meanings of personal artwork for women living with cancer. *Creativity Research Journal, 20*(2), 211–220. https://doi.org/10.1080/10400410802060059

Richman, D. R. (1988). Cognitive psychotherapy through the career cycle. In W. Dryden & P. Trower (Eds.), *Developments in cognitive psychotherapy* (pp. 190–217). Sage.

Rapp, C. A. (1998). *The strengths model: Case management with people suffering from severe and persistent mental illness.* Oxford University Press.

Rhodes, S. D., & Hergenrather, K. C. (2007). Exploring undergraduate student attitudes toward persons with disabilities application of the disability social relationship scale. *Rehabilitation Counseling Bulletin, 50*(2), 66–75.

Saita, E., & Tramontano, M. (2018). Navigating the complexity of the therapeutic and clinical use of photography in psychosocial settings: A review of the literature. *Research in Psychotherapy, 21*, 1–11.

Sayed, M. A. (2003). Conceptualization of mental illness within Arab cultures: Meeting challenges in cross-cultural settings. *Social behaviour and Personality, 31*, 333.

Sarbin, T. (1986). *Narrative psychology.* Praeger.

Savickas, M. L. (1991). The meaning of love and work: Career issues and interventions. *Career Development Quarterly, 39*, 315–324.

Schultheiss, D. P. (2000). Emotional-social issues in the provision of career counselling. In D. A. Luzzo (Ed.), *Career counselling of college students* (pp. 43–59). American Psychological Association.

Schudson, K. R. (1975). The simple camera in school counseling. *Personnel & Guidance Journal, 54*(4), 225–226. Retrieved from EBSCOhost.

Sharf, R. S. (2006). *Applying career development throey to counselling.* Thomas Wadsworth.

Swartz, L. (2002). *Culture and mental health: A South African view.* Oxford University Press.

Sodi, T., Mudhovozi, P., Mashamba, T., Radzalani-Makatu, M., Takalani, J., & Mabunda, J. (2011). Indigenous healing practices in the Limpopo Province of South Africa: A qualitative study. *International Journal of Health Promotion & Education, 49*, 101–110.

Sow, A. I. (1980). *Anthropological structures of madness in Black Africa.* International Universities Press.

Spiro, A. M. (2005). Najar of bhut – Evil eye or ghost affliction: Gujarati views about illness causation. *Anthropology & Medicine, 12*, 61–73.

Star, K. L., & Cox, J. A. (2008). The use of phototherapy in couples andfamily counseling. *Journal of Creativity in Mental Health, 3*(4), 373–382. https://doi.org/10.1080/15401380802527472

Sue, D. W., Bernier, J. B., Duran, M., Feinberg, L., Pedersen, P., et al. (1982). Position paper: Cross-cultural counselling competencies. *The Counseling Psychologist, 10*(2), 45–52.

Sue, D. W., Arredondo, P., & McDavis, R. (1992). Multicultural counseling competencies and standards: A call to the profession. *Journal of Counseling and Development, 70*, 477–486.

Sue, S., Zane, N., Nagayama Hall, G. C., & Berger, L. K. (2009a). The case for cultural competency in psychotherapeutic interventions. *Annual Review of Psychology, 60*, 525–548. https://doi.org/10.1146/annurev.psych.60.110707.163651

Sue, S., et al. (2009b). *Culturally responsive assessment questions for CBT+*. Retrieved from https://www.dcyf.wa.gov/sites/default/files/pdf/CulturallyResponsiveQuestions.pdf

Truter, I. (2007). African traditional healers: Cultural and religious beliefs intertwined in a holistic approach. *South African Pharmaceutical Journal, 74*, 56–60.

Uhrig, M. K., Trautmann, N., Baumgärtner, U., Treede, R.-D., Henrich, F., Hiller, W., & Marschall, S. (2016). Emotion elicitation: A comparison of pictures and films. *Frontiers in Psychology, 7*, 180. https://doi.org/10.3389/fpsyg.2016.00180

Weiser, J. (2004a). Photo Therapy techniques in counseling and therapy: Using ordinary snapshots and photo-interactions to help clients heal their lives. *The Canadian Art Therapy Association Journal, Fall, 17*(2), 23–53.

Weiser, J. (2004b). The continuum of arts-based healing practices: Arts-in-Therapy/Arts-asTherapy. Creative Arts in Counselling Chapter Newsletter (Canadian Counselling Association), Fall, *1*(2), 3.

Wessels, D. T. (1985). Using family photographs in the treatment of eating disorders. *Psychotherapy in Private Practice, 3*(4), 95–105.

Wilber, K. (2000). Integral Psychology. Boston, MA: Shambhala.

Young, R. A. (2001). *7¾? notion ofproject in vocational psychology*. Paper presented to the symposium "future directions in vocational psychology," at the annual convention of the Canadian Psychological Association, Laval University, Quebec.

Young, R. A., & Valach, L. (1996). Interpretation and action in career counseling. In M. L. Savickas & W. B. Walsh (Eds.), *Handbook of career counseling theory and practice* (pp. 361–375). Davies-Black.

Zalaquett, C. P., Fuerth, K. M., Stein, C., Ivey, A. E., & Ivey, M. B. (2008). Reframing the DSM-IV-TR from a multicultural/social justice perspective. *Journal of Counseling & Development, 86*, 364–371. https://doi.org/10.1002/j.1556-678.2008.tb00521.x

# Chapter 9
# Towards Well-being: Self-Care in the Supervisory Space

## 9.1 Introduction

Health professionals are trained to be caring and compassionate but also to set appropriate boundaries with clients or patients. Guy (2000) referred to this as working in a context of one-way caring, as we do not expect the same levels of caring and compassion in return. At the same time, establishing a therapeutic alliance and maintaining boundaries takes effort and energy, which could potentially be draining and impact negatively on our well-being (Skovholt & Trotter-Mathison, 2011). Further, working in resource-constrained contexts and specifically in the field of trauma may exacerbate the emotional burden of being a health professional (Posluns & Gall, 2020). Practitioners who prioritise self-care seem to be less at risk to experience negative outcomes such as burnout and traumatic stress (Butler et al., 2017). In addition, there is increasing evidence that self-care not only prevents stress but can enhance professional and personal well-being (Rupert & Dorociak, 2019). It is therefore imperative to consider how health professionals' self-care can be supported and enhanced in the supervisory space. This chapter provides an overview of the domains of self-care and proposes self-care strategies associated with these domains. The discussion is embedded in the framework of positive psychology, maintaining that self-care should not only aim to diminish negative outcomes but also enable mental health practitioners to flourish both personally and professionally (see also Mills, 2021; Wise et al., 2012).

---

This chapter was contributed by Prof. Catharina Guse.

K. V. Rawatlal, *Clinical Supervision in South Africa*, SpringerBriefs in Psychology, https://doi.org/10.1007/978-3-031-41929-4_9

## 9.2    What Is Self-Care?

Despite increased research and practical attention, there is no commonly agreed-upon definition of self-care (Wong & White, 2021). Earlier conceptualisations referred to actions that reduce the negative consequences of health professionals' work, for example, behaviours that '...lessen the amount of stress, anxiety, or emotional reaction experienced when working with clients' (Williams et al. 2010, p. 322). Other definitions also include a focus on positive functioning, describing self-care as a '...multidimensional, multifaceted process of purposeful engagement in strategies that promote healthy functioning and enhance well-being' (Dorociak et al., 2017, p.326), and 'engagement in behaviours that maintain and promote physical and emotional wellbeing' (Meyers al. 2012, p. 56). Self-care requires action and conscious effort, in addition to having resources available (Collins & Cassill, 2022; Colman et al. 2016; Pakenham, 2017).

Self-care has a relational component as it entails caring for ourselves in addition to caring for the others, i.e. clients, patients, or the therapeutic process (Butler et al., 2019; Kissil & Niño, 2017). Some scholars argued that the notion of self-care should move away from only considering individual practices and personal agency in initiating self-care. Rather, self-care should be a shared and reciprocal practice of being valued and caring with others (Lewis et al., 2022). This may be particularly important in training and supervision contexts where others could be supervisors, mentors, and colleagues. Self-care is also a 'way of being' (Mason, 2016, p.98), as both our interactions with clients and self-care activities can be meaningful tasks in their own right. Some authors view self-care as an essential professional competency that ensures effective professional functioning (Wise & Reuman, 2019) as well as an ethical obligation towards clients (Collins & Cassill, 2022; Mason, 2016; Ziede & Norcross, 2020).

In addition to these definitions, Butler et al. (2019) identified two main aims of self-care: First, to prevent negative outcomes, for example, stress, burnout, and compassion fatigue. Specifically, self-care is practised to '...guard against, cope with, or reduce stress and related adverse consequences' (p. 107). The second aim of practicing self-care is to strengthen or promote positive outcomes through maintaining and promoting well-being in the broadest sense. Therefore, self-care should inspire health professionals to aspire to the positive end of the continuum – reaching flourishing and not only averting the negative (Butler et al., 2019; Wise et al., 2012).

In this chapter, self-care is conceptualised broadly to include intentional strategies which we can implement to reduce the potential adverse effects of practising as a health care professional, as well as to promote well-being and flourishing. In other words, self-care is viewed as more than surviving and maintaining existing functioning, but also includes sustainable, meaningful activities that can be integrated into our daily lives and support optimal functioning (Wise & Reuman, 2019; Wise et al., 2012).

## 9.3  Why Focus on Self-Care?

Literature on self-care reported outcomes related to two main areas: prevention of negative outcomes and promotion of positive outcomes. In terms of negative outcomes, research has focused on the role of self-care in addressing the stress inherent to the work of a health care professional. Findings suggest that self-care is an important mechanism to reduce stress, leading to less burnout in practicing psychologists (Rupert & Dorociak, 2019), and also supported nurses' mental health during the COVID-19 pandemic (Lewis et al., 2022). Second, engaging in self-care promotes positive outcomes such as life satisfaction (Rupert & Dorociak, 2019) and general flourishing (Wise et al., 2012).

Considering the benefits of self-care for trainee health professionals, Myers et al. (2012) reported that self-care strategies such as utilising social support and cognitive reappraisal were linked with lower levels of perceived stress. Similarly, a meta-analysis indicated that self-care was associated with increased self-compassion and life satisfaction, as well as decreased anxiety and psychological distress among trainee psychologists (Colman et al., 2016). Importantly, self-care seems to be more effective when implemented intentionally and proactively to prevent negative outcomes, rather than addressing them once they occur (Posluns & Gall, 2020; Rupert & Dorociak, 2019). In other words, it may be less helpful to only address self-care needs when experiencing burnout or extreme stress. Overall, it is evident that implementing sustained, proactive strategies are important to health professionals' personal and professional well-being. As Butler et al. (2019, p. 107) stated, self-care is 'essential for the good of the therapist, the therapy, and the client'.

## 9.4  Domains and Strategies of Self-Care

Over the years, several scholars have provided guidelines and suggestions for effective self-care. These range from broad strategies (Norcross, 2000; Ziede & Norcross, 2020) to activities within specific areas of functioning (Posluns & Gall, 2020). While the aforementioned mostly focus on qualified health care professionals, there is also increased literature on integrating self-care in the training of health professionals (Collins & Cassill, 2022; Mills, 2021). Butler et al. (2019) proposed six domains of self-care which serve as a useful framework to identify areas and strategies that can be tailored to individual needs. These are the physical, professional, relational, emotional, psychological and spiritual domains. The sections that follow discuss these domains, integrating strategies from the field of positive psychology where relevant.

## 9.4.1  Physical Domain

Butler et al. (2019) viewed physical self-care as the foundation for all areas of healthy functioning. This domain is about taking care of our physical and bodily needs to support our well-being. Yet, Ziede and Norcross (2020) argued that we tend to ignore how central our bodies are to self-care. Taking care of the physical domain involves attending to sleep, nutrition, exercise, and maintaining health care.

*Sleep* is rejuvenating and essential to physical health. Strategies to promote good sleep include maintaining a regular sleep schedule and self-monitoring sleep habits (Posluns & Gall, 2020). Although trainee health professionals may be burning the proverbial midnight oil sporadically, getting sufficient sleep every night should be a prerogative.

*Nutrition* involves following a well-balanced diet that includes a variety of food groups and limiting sugar, saturated fats, salt highly processed foods (Butler et al., 2019). Proper hydration, hydration, i.e. drinking enough water, is equally as important to maintain physical health (Rokach & Boulazreg, 2022; Ziede & Norcross, 2020).

*Exercise* is essential to physical and psychological well-being, both by preventing ill-being and as a therapeutic intervention (Posluns & Gall, 2020; Walsh, 2011). Integrating exercise as part of self-care can start simply by aiming to be more active each day or by following structured exercise regimes like spinning classes or engaging in team sports. According to Zhang and Chen (2019), even as little as 10 min a day could increase subjective well-being. Being physically active enhances positive mood and affect, thus building psychological resources, which are vital to self-care (Hogan et al., 2015).

*Health maintenance* involves taking care of our physical and mental health through attending check-ups, monitoring symptoms, and adhering to existing treatment plans (Butler et al., 2019).

## 9.4.2  Professional Domain

Self-care in the professional domain addresses issues related to work. Professional self-care is about managing work-related stress, reducing the risk of burnout, and increasing work satisfaction and performance (Butler et al., 2019). In this domain, self-care starts with knowledge of the occupational hazards we may face, which, according to Zinn (2022) is essential self-care knowledge. Similarly, these hazards include a) burnout and job stress; b) vulnerability to secondary traumatic stress, vicarious traumatisation, and compassion fatigue; c) patient behaviours; and d) physical and emotional isolation.

### 9.4.2.1   Burnout

The nature of a career in the health professions involves exposure to numerous psychosocial stressors, which could lead to job stress and burnout (Rokach & Boulazreg, 2022). Burnout is characterised by physical, emotional, and mental exhaustion, due to working in emotionally demanding work contexts (Shaufeli & Greenglass, 2001). Much research has focused on the incidence of burnout in health professionals, with one study finding that 49% of trainee psychologists reported burnout (Kaeding et al., 2017). It is important to point out that burnout is not simply due to the environment, or the vulnerability of the person. Rather, it flows from the interaction between the person and the environment, which implies that health professionals need to work through their reactions and assumptions related to their work context (Ziede & Norcross, 2020). Since burnout among health professionals is more difficult to address than work stress (Dreison et al., 2018), it is essential that we identify and attend to work stressors before it leads to burnout.

### 9.4.2.2   Vulnerability to Secondary Traumatic Stress, Vicarious Traumatisation and Compassion Fatigue

A large part of health professionals' work may involve assisting clients who have experienced trauma. This may lead to secondary traumatisation, which is a stress response that occurs due to being compassionate and empathetic towards a traumatised person and includes symptoms associated with post-traumatic stress disorder (Figley, 2002; Knight, 2013). Related to this, vicarious traumatisation may occur due to working with traumatised clients over an extended period. Butler et al. (2019) indicated that vicarious traumatisation can have a detrimental effect on health professionals' identity, perceptions of the world, beliefs, psychological needs, and memories. Finally, we may also be vulnerable to compassion fatigue. Symptoms of compassion fatigue are similar to those of secondary traumatisation but are characterised by a diminished ability to care for clients. This is a consequence of being exposed to clients' suffering and trauma over an extended period (Cavanagh et al., 2020).

### 9.4.2.3   Patient Behaviours

Individuals visit health care professionals because they experience some form of distress. Unfortunately, this means that we may be exposed to intense emotional displays as well as severe mental health problems (Rokach & Boulazreg, 2022). For example, psychologists view suicidal ideation, suicidal acts, aggression directed towards the psychologist, premature termination, and extreme apathy and depression as the most distressing patient behaviours (Ziede & Norcross, 2020). Health professionals should be prepared for the potentially disruptive effects of such behaviours on their personal and professional lives.

#### 9.4.2.4   Physical and Emotional Isolation

While we need to ensure privacy and confidentiality for our clients, working in a consulting room for hours on end puts us at risk for environmental deprivation. Further, we have to set aside our own emotional concerns, which may lead to feeling lonely and emotionally isolated (Rokach & Boulazreg, 2022; Ziede & Norcross, 2020).

Given these occupational hazards, it may be easy to think that it is inevitable for health professionals to experience burnout and intense work stress. However, knowing the hazards makes it possible to prevent negative consequences by practicing self-care preventatively. Strategies to implement work-related self-care include developing effective coping strategies, maintaining a healthy work-life balance, setting boundaries, utilising social support, and seeking supervision (Bressi & Vaden, 2017; Butler et al., 2019; Ziede & Norcross, 2020). Focusing on the rewards of the profession, as well as revisiting the personal values that led to this career choice, may be a useful strategy (Posluns & Gall, 2020; Ziede & Norcross, 2020). One such reward is compassion satisfaction, which follows having worked effectively with a client (Radey & Figley, 2007). Acknowledging successes and work-related strengths could support overall well-being over time (e.g. Meyers & van Woerkom, 2017; Wood et al., 2011). Activities such as journaling and making lists of what you are grateful for in your professional life can strengthen a focus on what is going well, rather than on only the hazards you may come across. Some of these strategies will be discussed in more detail in the sections to follow.

### 9.4.3   Relational Domain

This domain of self-care concerns relationships in the broadest sense. Butler et al. (2019) described relationship self-care as efforts to strengthen and maintain interpersonal bonds. This can range from close friends and family members, to work acquaintances and pets. Nurturing relationships with others in our lives is an important self-care activity, as having healthy close relationships is strongly linked to well-being (Gable, 2019). Relational self-care activities include utilising social support, nurturing close relationships, and engaging in acts of kindness.

#### 9.4.3.1   Social Support

Social support refers to resources provided by others, as well as interactions with others that help us cope in times of stress (Clark et al., 2009). Similarly, perceived social support is the belief that others will be there for you during difficult times in the future (Cohen & Wills, 1985). Having and utilising social support networks protect against the emotional impact of stressors and is essential to self-care. Social support networks can be professional (e.g. peers, supervisors, colleagues, and mentors) or personal (family members, partners, close friends, personal therapy) in nature. Research indicates that professional support is particularly important to the well-being of trainee clinical psychologists, being associated with increased flourishing and positive affect, and decreased perceived stress and negative affect (Zahniser et al., 2017). It is essential that we utilise sources of available support intentionally to reap the benefits thereof.

### 9.4.3.2   Nurturing Close Relationships

This strategy involves being mindful of and prioritising relationships with important others. Responding with emotional fondness (Gable & Reis, 2010) and expressing gratitude in the relationship (Algoe, 2012; Leong et al., 2020) are two strategies that can strengthen relationships, thereby enhancing social support and well-being. Relational savouring, where we consciously pay attention to positive relational experiences can also strengthen relationships (Guse, 2020). Research suggests that spending time with family, close friends, and/or partners is the most important self-care strategy for trainee psychologists and qualified professionals (Ziede & Norcross, 2020). Therefore, it may be wise to explicitly address this domain in developing a self-care plan.

### 9.4.3.3   Acts of Kindness

These are altruistic behaviours towards others that can strengthen interpersonal connections and increase well-being (Guse, 2020; Ko et al., 2021). These acts need not be on a large scale but can be as simple as helping a colleague with a task, bringing a meal to a sick neighbour, or paying for someone's coffee. Research increasingly indicates that altruistic acts benefit both the receiver and the person who enacts kindness. One of the important benefits of altruistic acts is that it leads to an increase in positive emotions in the present (see also sect. 4.4) which strengthens psychological resources and supports well-being (Curry et al., 2018; Pressman et al., 2015).

## *9.4.4   Emotional Domain*

Butler et al. (2019) differentiated emotional self-care from relationship self-care, defining it as '… practices that are engaged in to safeguard against or address negative emotional experience as well as those intended to create or enhance positive emotional experience and well-being' (p. 114). Here the two aims of self-care are aligned: to minimise negative outcomes and to promote well-being through attending to our emotional experiences. The first involves addressing destructive coping styles and reducing negative emotional experiences, while the second is about strategies to enhance positive emotions.

### 9.4.4.1   Destructive Ways of Coping: Reflect and Replace

We all have preferred strategies and ways of coping. Are these still working and conducive to your overall well-being? Self-care in this domain is about identifying those coping skills that may not be conducive in the long term, such as using alcohol and caffeine, binge eating, spending money, watching television, or ignoring personal distress (Burgess et al., 2010; Butler et al., 2019). We need to be mindful of when we use strategies that seem helpful in the short term but are not sustainable over time. Also, replacing destructive coping strategies with ones that build personal psychological resources is central to self-care.

### 9.4.4.2   Reducing Negative Emotional Experience

This involves general strategies to counter negative emotional experiences, such as mindfulness meditation, yoga, relaxation exercises, and self-hypnosis (Butler et al., 2019). Psychologists often recommend such evidence-based strategies to clients to reduce emotional distress, so it is only apt for health professionals to similarly implement them in their own lives as well.

### 9.4.4.3   Increasing Positive Emotions

This strategy is about using activities that elicit positivity and feelings of happiness and well-being. Experiencing positive emotions can build psychological resources and contribute to an upward spiral of well-being over time (Fredrickson & Joiner, 2002). It is important to note that increasing positive emotions is not simply about just feeling more pleasure. Rather, when we experience positive emotions we can generate more possible routes of action through increased cognitive awareness. In turn, we can take in more information that assists us in building resilience, strengthening our relationships, and coping with difficult situations (Fredrickson, 2013; Waters et al., 2022), making it essential to self-care. Activities that can increase positive emotions include savouring, loving-kindness meditation, as well as practicing self-compassion and gratitude.

*Savouring* occurs when we intentionally focus on forgotten or neglected positive experiences (Stone & Parks, 2018). It is possible to enhance the experience of remembering pleasant experiences from the past, attending to positive emotions in the present experience, or anticipating a pleasant future event and the positive emotions that it may evoke. What is essential is that one should be aware of positive feelings during these experiences, and also manage and regulate the positive experience (Bryant, 2021; Guse, 2020). This implies slowing down, attending to, and appreciating positive experiences in your life, which can range from sensory pleasures such as eating a special meal, to being in nature and sharing special moments with loved ones.

*Loving-Kindness Meditation (LKM)* aims to increase positive emotions such as feelings of warmth and caring towards self and others. It has a strong focus on the context of interpersonal relationships (Fredrickson, 2009; Fredrickson et al., 2017). LKM intends to develop love for others rather than only elicit awareness in the present moment. This love extends beyond close friends and family to all living beings (Stone & Parks, 2018). One way of practicing LKM is by repeating statements such as the following statements: 'May this one (or I, they, we) be safe' / 'May they be happy. /May they be healthy' LKM has been proposed as a strategy to reduce stress and implicit bias in health professionals (Murphy et al., 2023), with evidence of its stress-reducing effect reported among nursing professionals (Mulianda et al., 2022) and increased empathy in student counsellors (Leppma & Young, 2016). Given that LKM also leads to sustained well-being in the long term (Cohn & Fredrickson, 2010), it is a sustainable self-care strategy that could easily be incorporated into everyday life (Wise et al., 2012).

*Practicing self-compassion* entails creating and nurturing a caring and warm relationship with the self (Neff, 2003) and can be viewed as a positive emotion that supports self-care (Mills, 2021). It involves extending the same kindness and compassion to oneself that one would offer to others during difficult times (Germer, 2009; Neff, 2011). Further, practicing self-compassion enables a healthy way of relating to oneself when experiencing personal failures or negative life events, balancing our strengths with challenges that comes our way (Neff, 2003; Neff & Lamb, 2009). As health professionals, it may be easier to direct compassion to our clients than to ourselves, which is why intentional self-compassion is an important aspect of self-care. Existing research suggests that self-compassion is linked to increased self-care and professional quality of life, as well as a decrease in perceived burnout risk and secondary traumatic stress among health professionals (Garcia et al., 2021). Self-compassion also predicts self-care (Jay Miller et al., 2019). Therefore, professionals who practice more self-compassion may be more likely to actively engage in activities that would promote self-care.

*Practicing gratitude* is about being focused on the present, being grateful for your life as it is at this moment, and being thankful to what and who has contributed to it (Lyubomirsky, 2008). The intentional practice of gratitude can trigger the experience of positive emotions and thus increase well-being. The most common ways of practicing gratitude are gratitude journaling, writing a gratitude letter, and writing down three good things that happened in a day (Jans-Beken et al., 2020). Gratitude journaling involves regularly writing about things, events and people we are grateful for (Kaczmarek et al., 2015; Parks et al., 2012). The gratitude letter requires the individual to write a letter to someone they have not properly thanked and deliver (and preferably read) it in person (Seligman et al., 2006). Writing down three good things (Lai & O'Carroll, 2017; Seligman et al., 2005) is similar to journaling, but is a more structured exercise where one writes down what one is thankful for during a specific period, for example, once or twice a week or even daily. It is important to take time to reflect when writing journaling or writing gratitude lists to maximise the benefits thereof (Guse, 2020). Research indicates that gratitude activities lead to increases in positive affect, life satisfaction, and well-being, as well as decreased stress (Lai & O'Carroll, 2017; Meyer & Stutts, 2023). Studies among health care professionals reported that engaging in gratitude practice increased self-care behaviours and coping self-efficacy (Caragol et al., 2022), improved stress management, and supported overall well-being (Adair et al., 2020; Cumella, 2022). Since gratitude activities are relatively simple to implement and may rather quickly improve mood, they can be easily incorporated into a daily self-care plan.

### 9.4.5　Psychological Domain

Butler et al. (2019, p. 116) describe self-care in the psychological domain as '…concerning the life of the mind and experience of self'. It is about purposefully understanding, and attending to, the intellectual and overall needs of the self. The following areas of psychological self-care will be discussed in this section: self-awareness, practicing mindfulness, and engaging in other intellectual pursuits that are inherently enjoyable.

*Self-awareness* involves noticing and reflecting on our internal and external experiences. Noticing when we feel drained opens up avenues to take steps to replenish resources and can strengthen our self-care plan (Butler et al., 2019; Posluns & Gall, 2020; Sansó et al. 2015). Further, practicing self-awareness can help to maintain positive feelings about work when experiencing high stress levels (Rupert & Dorociak, 2019). Self-awareness can be increased through monitoring ourselves using questionnaires related to domains of self-care (Butler et al., 2019), journaling about experiences and reflections (Ziede & Norcross, 2020), as well as engaging in personal psychotherapy and supervision (Butler et al., 2019; Posluns & Gall, 2020).

*Mindfulness* is about purposefully paying attention to what is happening in the moment in a non-judgemental manner, noticing how experience unfolds moment by moment (Kabat-Zinn, 2003). However, mindfulness can also be moments of stillness and peace, even when busy with other things, thereby regaining contact with being by reminding yourself to be mindful (Kabat-Zinn, 2009). In mindfulness meditation, we focus attention to observe our conscious attention in the present moment, holding an open and accepting attitude, broadening our conscious experience (Fredrickson et al., 2017). There is substantive research evidence for the conducive effect of mindfulness meditation on the experience of well-being. For example, Ivtzan & Lomas (2016) reported increases in positive emotions, self-compassion, happiness, meaning, and compassion, as well as decreases in stress and depression, which were still present after 1 month of the intervention. Butler et al. (2019) proposed that mindfulness, particularly when adopted as a way of being, can cultivate self-awareness and greater clarity on personal experiences, which is important to self-care. Practitioners can easily integrate mindfulness into everyday life by purposefully initiating brief mindfulness pauses throughout the day (Rokach & Boulazreg, 2019).

*Intellectual and enjoyable pursuits of the mind* include cognitive activities that provide a respite from everyday stressors, for example, poetry, cinema, reading, playing games, and solving puzzles (Butler et al., 2019). Ziede and Norcross (2020, p. 600) also refer to engaging in 'healthy escapes' such as hobbies, going on vacations, and using humour to deal with stress. It is important to make time for these pleasures regularly and direct attention away from professional experiences. This supports us to maintain balance among different life domains, which is an important area of self-care (Posluns & Gall, 2020).

### 9.4.6 Spiritual Domain

This domain of self-care involves how we make sense of our place in the world and foster connections to something larger than the self. Butler et al. (2019) proposed that it is about finding hope, purpose, and meaning in life. They continued to define spiritual self-care as deeply personal and a practice that '… creates space to reflect on our own inner needs and our role or place within the world and universe' (p. 118). Spirituality encompasses more than religion and entails connections with self, others, and the divine, in addition to purpose and meaning (Pargament, 1999). According to Butler et al. (2019), spiritual self-care can be based either on faith-based practice or secular practice.

*Faith-based spirituality* includes participating in organised religion or engaging in prayer. Religion is important to the lives of many individuals and several studies have reported a positive association between religious practice and well-being (see Graham & Newman, 2018, for an overview). It has further been linked to better coping during stressful times, such as the recent pandemic (Thomas & Barbato, 2020) while participating in religious activities showed a significant relationship with mental health (Garssen et al., 2021). Prayer is a common practice in many religions. It is an attempt to establish a connection with the divine, with strong contemplative elements (Bradshaw & Kent, 2018; Butler et al., 2019). In several religions, gratitude is practiced as prayer, consequently supporting well-being (see also sect. xx for the benefits of gratitude). For religious health professionals, practicing their religion can therefore support self-care.

*Secular spirituality* comprises a search for meaning independent of religious institutions and doctrines. It also '… highly values one's relationship with the self, others, nature, life's meaning, and transcendence or sense of the ultimate' (Sperry, 2016, p. 221). Several practices can strengthen this broader experience of spirituality, while meditative practice, specifically spiritual meditation and transcendental meditation (Bonamer and Aquino-Russell 2019; Butler et al., 2019), can enhance self-care. An additional strategy is to actively practice meaning-making, which involves contextualising stressors within one's overall values and belief system, revisiting one's purpose of working in the health professions field, and connecting with the transcendent meaning of one's work (Park, 2010; Posluns & Gall, 2020). Finally, experiences in nature can contribute to spiritual self-care by providing time to reflect and heal. This includes going for walks, camping, or gardening. Research suggests that spending time in nature is associated with better physical health and well-being (Oh et al., 2017; White et al. 2019) and could be considered a sustainable self-care activity when integrated into daily life.

## 9.5    Self-Care in the Supervisory Context

The central theme of this book concerns the supervision of health professionals. The supervisory context provides an important space to model, monitor, support, and encourage self-care (Colman et al., 2016). Students in the health professions may face difficulty in balancing academic, clinical, and personal demands. It is important to prioritise their well-being in addition to meeting the academic outcomes of professional training (Mills, 2021). Given that they have limited professional experience, it is imperative that training and supervision intentionally and strategically emphasise and support self-care (Collins & Cassill, 2022).

In the professional domain of self-care, supervisors can assist by acknowledging the nature of the health profession and being open to discussing possible risks the supervisee may encounter (Posluns & Gall, 2020). Students in the health care professions are prone to experiencing traumatisation and secondary traumatic stress due to being exposed to stress and trauma during their practicum (Butler et al., 2019). This may be even more evident in resource-constrained contexts where they have to deal with complex cases as there are limited opportunities for referrals to more experienced practitioners. Without this knowledge, they will not be able to identify areas of concern or act to remedy these areas. Supervisors, therefore, have an important role in discussing signs of burnout and stress with their supervisees (Collins & Cassill, 2022). Further related to the professional domain of self-care, supervisees often use supervision to discuss ethical dilemmas and concerns. Engaging in self-care is an ethical obligation, since a lack of self-care may lead to harming the client and lead to unethical practice (Mason, 2016; Posluns & Gall, 2020).

Supervision also involves the relational domain of self-care, as supervisors serve as an important source of social support (Posluns & Gall, 2020). An emotionally safe supervisory space that offers an opportunity to reflect on experiences with clients is essential to supporting trainees' self-care and professional development.

In the emotional domain of self-care, supervisors can monitor trainees' coping strategies and suggest activities to practice self-care. It is well-known that younger mental health care professionals are inclined to demonstrate lower levels of self-care and self-compassion (Jay Miller et al., 2019). Supervisors can support supervisees' self-care and self-compassion by encouraging skills development in these areas and modelling self-care in the supervisory relationship.

The supervisory space provides an essential context to engage in self-awareness, which is a key aspect of psychological self-care. Reflective supervision (Glassburn et al., 2019) can support high-quality professional services, and at the same time support trainees to examine their practical experiences and identify areas for professional development and self-care. Acknowledgement of supervisees' strengths and successes could further support self-care in this domain and facilitate a state of flourishing versus only surviving the demands of professional training (see also Wise et al., 2012).

Despite an increase in literature on the importance of self-care for health professionals in general, and mental health professions specifically, professional training programmes may not adequately address self-care (Bamonti et al., 2014). This may be equally true of supervision. Training programs can play an important role in cultivating an attitude of self-care for students in mental health professions (Posluns & Gall, 2020). It is also essential that self-care is not only considered for trainees who are at risk or currently are experiencing difficulty in managing the demands of training. Rather, engaging in continuous self-care practices should be encouraged as key to overall well-being (Bamonti et al. 2014).

## 9.6   Conclusion

Caring for others is at the heart of being a health professional. This chapter discussed the importance of self-care for trainees and provided suggestions for self-care strategies in six domains of self-care. Supervision is a central context through which self-care can be supported and developed. I hope that professional training and supervision can be a space where strengths are celebrated, and reflection becomes a source of meaning and personal growth. Ultimately, practicing consistent, sustainable self-care as health professionals can lead to thriving, not just surviving.

## References

Adair, K. C., Rodriguez-Homs, L. G., Masoud, S., Mosca, P. J., & Sexton, J. B. (2020). Gratitude at work: Prospective cohort study of a web-based, single-exposure well-being intervention for health care workers. *Journal of Medical Internet Research, 22*(5), e15562.

Algoe, S. B. (2012). Find, remind, and bind: The functions of gratitude in everyday relationships. *Social and Personality Psychology Compass, 6*(6), 455–469.

Bamonti, P. M., Keelan, C. M., Larson, N., Mentrikoski, J. M., Randall, C. L., Sly, S. K., et al. (2014). Promoting ethical behavior by cultivating a culture of self-care during graduate training: A call to action. *Training and Education in Professional Psychology, 8*(4), 253.

Bonamer, J. R., & Aquino-Russell, C. (2019). Self-care strategies for professional development: Transcendental meditation reduces compassion fatigue and improves resilience for nurses. *Journal for Nurses in Professional Development, 35*(2), 93–97.

Bradshaw, M., & Kent, B. V. (2018). Prayer, attachment to God, and changes in psychological well-being in later life. *Journal of Aging and Health, 30*(5), 667–691.

Bressi, S. K., & Vaden, E. R. (2017). Reconsidering self care. *Clinical Social Work Journal, 45*(1), 33–38. https://doi.org/10.1007/s10615-016-0575-4

Bryant, F. B. (2021). Current progress and future directions for theory and research on savoring. *Frontiers in Psychology, 12*, 771698.

Burgess, L., Irvine, F., & Wallymahmed, A. (2010). Personality, stress and coping in intensive care nurses: A descriptive exploratory study. *Nursing in Critical Care, 15*(3), 129–140.

Butler, L. D., Carello, J., & Maguin, E. (2017). Trauma, stress, and self-care in clinical training: Predictors of burnout, decline in health status, secondary traumatic stress symptoms, and compassion satisfaction. *PsychologicalTrauma: Theory, Research, Practice, and Policy, 9*(4), 416–424. https://doi.org/10.1037/tra0000187

Butler, L. D., Mercer, K. A., McClain-Meeder, K., Horne, D. M., & Dudley, M. (2019). Six domains of self-care: Attending to the whole person. *Journal of Human Behavior in the Social Environment, 29*(1), 107–124.

Caragol, J. A., Johnson, A. R., & Kwan, B. M. (2022). A gratitude intervention to improve clinician stress and professional satisfaction: A pilot and feasibility trial. *The International Journal of Psychiatry in Medicine, 57*(2), 103–116.

Cavanagh, N., Cockett, G., Heinrich, C., Doig, L., Fiest, K., Guichon, J. R., et al. (2020). Compassion fatigue in healthcare providers: A systematic review and meta-analysis. *Nursing Ethics, 27*(3), 639–665.

Clark, H. K., Murdock, N. L., & Koetting, K. (2009). Predicting burnout and career choice satisfaction in counseling psychology graduate students. *The Counseling Psychologist, 37*(4), 580–606.

Cohen, S., & Wills, T. A. (1985). Stress, social support, and the stress buffering hypothesis. *Psychological Bulletin, 98*, 310–357. https://doi.org/10.1037/0033-2909.98.2.310

Cohn, M. A., & Fredrickson, B. L. (2010). In search of durable positive psychology interventions: Predictors and consequences of long-term positive behavior change. *Journal of Positive Psychology, 5*, 355–366. https://doi.org/10.1080/17439760.2010.508883

Collins, M. H., & Cassill, C. K. (2022). Psychological wellness and self-care: An ethical and professional imperative. *Ethics & Behavior, 32*(7), 634–646.

Colman, D. E., Echon, R., Lemay, M. S., McDonald, J., Smith, K. R., Spencer, J., & Swift, J. K. (2016). The efficacy of self-care for graduate students in professional psychology: A meta-analysis. *Training and Education in Professional Psychology, 10*(4), 188–197. https://doi.org/10.1037/tep0000130

Cumella, K. (2022). Gratitude journals can improve nurses' mental well-being. *Nursing, 52*(12), 58–61.

Curry, O. S., Rowland, L. A., Van Lissa, C. J., Zlotowitz, S., McAlaney, J., & Whitehouse, H. (2018). Happy to help? A systematic review and meta-analysis of the effects of performing acts of kindness on the well-being of the actor. *Journal of Experimental Social Psychology, 76*, 320–329. https://doi.org/10.1016/j.jesp.2018.02.014

Dorociak, K. E., Rupert, P. A., Bryant, F. B., & Zahniser, E. (2017). Development of professional self-care scale. *Journal of Counseling Psychology, 64*(3), 325–334. https://doi.org/10.1037/cou0000206

Dreison, K. C., Luther, L., Bonfils, K. A., Sliter, M. T., McGrew, J. H., Salyers, M. P., et al. (2018). Job burnout in mental health providers: A meta-analysis of 35 years of intervention research. *Journal of Occupational Health Psychology, 23*(1), 18–30. https://doi.org/10.1037/ocp0000047

Figley, C. R. (2002). Compassion fatigue: Psychotherapists' chronic lack of self care. *Psychotherapy in Practice, 58*(11), 1433–1441.

Fredrickson, B. L. (2009). *Positivity*. Crown Publishers.

Fredrickson, B. L. (2013). Positive emotions broaden and build. In P. Devine & A. Plant (Eds.), *Advances in experimental social psychology* (Vol. 47, pp. 1–53). Academic. https://doi.org/10.1016/B978-0-12-407236-7.00001-

Fredrickson, B. L., & Joiner, T. (2002). Positive emotions trigger upward spirals toward emotional well-being. *Psychological Science, 13*(2), 172–175.

Fredrickson, B. L., Boulton, A. J., Firestine, A. M., Van Cappellen, P., Algoe, S. B., Brantley, M. M., et al. (2017). Positive emotion correlates of meditation practice: A comparison of mindfulness meditation and loving-kindness meditation. *Mindfulness, 8*, 1623–1633. https://doi.org/10.1007/s12671-017-0735-9

Gable, S. L. (2019). Close relationships. In E. J. Finkel & R. F. Baumeister (Eds.), *Advanced social psychology: The state of the science* (2nd ed., pp. 227–247). Oxford University Press.

Gable, S. L., & Reis, H. T. (2010). Good news! Capitalizing on positive events in an interpersonal context. *Advances in Experimental Social Psychology, 42*, 195–257.

Garcia, A. C. M., Silva, B. D., da Silva, L. C. O., & Mills, J. (2021). Self-compassion in hospice and palliative care: A systematic integrative review. *Journal of Hospice & Palliative Nursing, 23*(2), 145–154.

Garssen, B., Visser, A., & Pool, G. (2021). Does spirituality or religion positively affect mental health? Meta-analysis of longitudinal studies. *The International Journal for the Psychology of Religion, 31*(1), 4–20.

Germer, C. K. (2009). *The mindful path to self-compassion.* Guilford Press.

Glassburn, S., & McGuire, L & Lay, K (2019). Reflection as self-care: models for facilitative supervision. Reflective Practice. 20. 1–13. https://doi.org/10.1080/14623943.2019.1674271

Guse, T. (2020). Activities and programmes to enhance well-being. In M. P. Wissing, J. C. Potgieter, T. Guse, I. P. Khumalo, & L. Nel (Eds.), *Towards flourishing: Embracing well-being in diverse contexts* (pp. 339–375). Van Schaik.

Guy, J. D. (2000). Self-care corner: Holding the holding environment together: Self-psychology and psychotherapist care. *Professional Psychology: Research and Practice, 31*(3), 351–352.

Hogan, C. L., Catalino, L. I., Mata, J., & Fredrickson, B. L. (2015). Beyond emotional benefits: Physical activity and sedentary behaviour affect psychosocial resources through emotions. *Psychology and Health, 30*, 354–369. https://doi.org/10.1080/08870446.2014.973410

Ivtzan, I., & Lomas, T. (2016). Mindfulness in positive psychology: the science of meditation and wellbeing. London: Routledge.

Jans-Beken, L., Jacobs, N., Janssens, M., Peeters, S., Reijnders, J., Lechner, L., & Lataster, J. (2020). Gratitude and health: An updated review. *Journal of Positive Psychology, 15*(6), 743–782. https://doi.org/10.1080/17439760.2019.1651888

Jay Miller, J., Lee, J., Niu, C., Grise-Owens, E., & Bode, M. (2019). Self-compassion as a predictor of self-care: A study of social work clinicians. *Clinical Social Work Journal, 47*, 321–331.

Kabat-Zinn, J. (2003). Mindfulness-based interventions in context: Past, present, and future. *Clinical Psychology: Science and Practice, 10*, 144–156. https://doi.org/10.1093/clipsy/bpg016

Kabat-Zinn, J. (2009). *Full catastrophe living: How to cope with stress, pain and illness using mindfulness meditation* (4th ed.).

Kaczmarek, L.D., Kashdan, T.B., Drazkowski, D., Enko, J., Kosakowski, M., Szaefer, A. & Bujacz, A. (2015). Why do people prefer gratitude journaling over gratitude letters? The influence of individual differences in motivation and personality on web-based interventions. Personality and Individual Differences, 75, 1–6. https://doi.org/https://doi.org/10.3389/fpsyg.2019.00584.

Kaeding, A., Sougleris, C., Reid, C., Vreeswijk, M. F., Hayes, C., Dorrian, J., & Simpson, S. (2017). Professional burnout, early maladaptive schemas, and physical health in clinical and counselling psychology trainees. *Journal of Clinical Psychology, 73*(12), 1782–1796. https://doi.org/10.1002/jclp.22485

Kissil, K., & Niño, A. (2017). Does the person-of-the-therapist training (POTT) promote self-care? Personal gains of MFT trainees following POTT: A retrospective thematic analysis. *Journal of Marital and Family Therapy, 43*(3), 526–536. https://doi.org/10.1111/jmft.12213

Knight, C. (2013). Indirect trauma: Implications for self-care, supervision, the organization, and the academic institution. *The Clinical Supervisor, 32*, 224–243. https://doi.org/10.1080/07325223.2013.850139

Ko, K., Margolis, S., Revord, J., & Lyubomirsky, S. (2021). Comparing the effects of performing and recalling acts of kindness. *Journal of Positive Psychology, 16*(1), 73–81. https://doi.org/10.1080/17439760.2019.1663252

Lai, S. T., & O'Carroll, R. E. (2017). "The three good things": The effects of gratitude practice in wellbeing: A randomised controlled trial. *Health Psychology Update, 26*, 10–18.

Leong, J. L. T., Chen, S. X., Fung, H. H. L., Bond, M. H., Siu, N. Y. F., & Zhu, J. Y. (2020). Is gratitude always beneficial to interpersonal relationships? The interplay of grateful disposition, grateful mood, and grateful expression among married couples. *Personality and Social Psychology Bulletin, 46*(1), 64–78. https://doi.org/10.1177/0146167219842868

Leppma, M., & Young, M. E. (2016). Loving-kindness meditation and empathy: A wellness group intervention for counseling students. *Journal of Counseling & Development, 94*(3), 297–305.

Lewis, S., Willis, K., Bismark, M., & Smallwood, N. (2022). A time for self-care? Frontline health workers' strategies for managing mental health during the COVID-19 pandemic. *SSM-Mental Health, 2*, 100053.

Lyubomirsky, S. (2008). *The how of happiness: A scientific approach to getting the life you want.* Penguin Books.

Mason, H. D. (2016). Logotherapeutic self-care. *The International Forum for Logotherapy, 39*, 97–102.

Meyer, H. H., & Stutts, L. A. (2023). The impact of single-session gratitude interventions on stress and affect. The Journal of Positive Psychology, 1–8. https://doi.org/https://doi.org/10.108 0/17439760.2023.2170823, 1.

Meyers, M. C., & Van Woerkom, M. (2017). Effects of a strengths intervention on general and work-related well-being: The mediating role of positive affect. *Journal of Happiness Studies, 18*, 671–689. https://doi.org/10.1007/s10902-016-9745-x

Mills, J. (2021). Theoretical foundations for self-care practice. *Progress in Palliative Care, 29*(4), 183–185.

Mulianda, D., Rahmanti, A., Margiyati, M., Sari, N. W., Haksara, E., & Pranata, S. (2022). Behavioral activation, mindfulness exercises, and loving-kindness meditation exercises as effective therapies to reduce stress among nursing students' during COVID-19 pandemic. *Open Access Macedonian Journal of Medical Sciences, 10*(G), 228–232.

Murphy, J., Farrell, K., Kealy, M. B., & Kristiniak, S. (2023). Mindfulness as a self-care strategy for healthcare professionals to reduce stress and implicit bias. *Journal of Interprofessional Education & Practice, 30*, 100598.

Myers, S. B., Sweeney, A. C., Popick, V., Wesley, K., Bordfeld, A., & Fingerhut, R. (2012). Self-care practices and perceived stress levels among psychology graduate students. *Training and Education in Professional Psychology, 6*(1), 55–66.

Neff, K. D. (2003). The development and validation of a scale to measure self-compassion. *Self and Identity, 2*(3), 223–250.

Neff, K. D. (2011). *Self-compassion.* William Morrow.

Neff, K. D., & Lamb, L. M. (2009). Self-compassion. In S. Lopez (Ed.), *The encyclopaedia of positive psychology* (pp. 864–867). Blackwell Publishing.

Newman, D. B., & Graham, J. (2018). Religion and well-being. In E. Diener, S. Oishi, & L. Tay (Eds.), Handbook of well-being. Salt Lake City, UT: DEF Publishers. DOI: HYPERLINK "http://nobascholar.com" nobascholar.com.

Norcross, J. C. (2000). Psychologist self-care: Practitioner-tested, research-informed strategies. *Professional Psychology: Research and Practice, 31*(6), 710–713. https://doi.org/10.1037/0735-7028.31.6.710

Oh, B., Lee, K. J., Zaslawski, C., Yeung, A., Rosenthal, D., Larkey, L., & Back, M. (2017). Health and Well-being benefits of spending time in forests: Systematic review. *Environmental Health and Preventive Medicine, 22*(1), 1–11.

Pakenham, K. I. (2017). Training in acceptance commitment therapy foster self-care in clinical psychology trainees. *Clinical Psychologist, 21*, 186–194. https://doi.org/10.1111/cp.12062

Pargament, K. I. (1999). The psychology of religion and spirituality?: Yes and no. *The International Journal for the Psychology of Religion, 9*, 3–16.

Park, C. L. (2010). Making sense of the meaning literature: An integrative review of meaning making and its effects on adjustment to stressful life events. *Psychological Bulletin, 136*(2), 257–301. https://doi.org/10.1037/a001830

Parks, A. C., Della Porta, M. D., Pierce, R. S., Zilca, R., & Lyubomirsky, S. (2012). Pursuing happiness in everyday life: The characteristics and behaviors of online happiness seekers. *Emotion, 12*(6), 1222.

Posluns, K., & Gall, T. L. (2020). Dear mental health practitioners, take care of yourselves: A literature review on self-care. *International Journal for the Advancement of Counselling, 42*, 1–20.

Pressman, S. D., Kraft, T. L., & Cross, M. P. (2015). It's good to do good and receive good: The impact of a "pay it forward" style kindness intervention on giver and receiver well-being. *Journal of Positive Psychology, 10*, 293–302. https://doi.org/10.1080/17439760.2014.965269

Radey, M., & Figley, C. R. (2007). The social psychology of compassion. *Clinical Social Work, 35*, 207–214. https://doi.org/10.1007/s10615-007-0087-3

Rokach, A. (2019) The Psychological Journey to and from Loneliness; Elsevier: Amsterdam, The Netherlands.

Rokach, A., Boulazreg, S. (2022). The COVID-19 era: How therapists can diminish burnout symptoms through self-care. *Curr Psychol 41*, 5660–5677. https://doi.org/10.1007/s12144-020-01149-6

Rupert, P. A., & Dorociak, K. E. (2019). Self-care, stress, and Well-being among practicing psychologists. *Professional Psychology: Research and Practice, 50*(5), 343.

Sansó, N., Galiana, L., Oliver, A., Pascual, A., Sinclair, S., & Benito, E. (2015). Palliative care professionals' inner life: Exploring the relationships among awareness, self-care, and compassion satisfaction and fatigue, burnout, and coping with death. *Journal of Pain and Symptom Management, 50*(2), 200–207.

Schaufeli, W.B. and Greenglass, E.R. (2001) Introduction to Special Issue on Burnout and Health. Psychology and Health, 16, 501–510. http://dx.doi.org/10.1080/08870440108405523

Seligman, M. E., Steen, T. A., Park, N., & Peterson, C. (2005). Positive psychology progress: Empirical validation of interventions. *American Psychologist, 60*(5), 410.

Seligman, M. E., Rashid, T., & Parks, A. C. (2006). Positive psychotherapy. *American Psychologist, 61*(8), 774.

Skovholt, T., & Trotter-Mathison, M. (2011). *The resilient practitioner: Burnout prevention and self-care strategies for counselors, therapists, teachers, and health professionals* (2nd ed.). Taylor & Francis.

Sperry, L. (2016). Secular spirituality and spiritually sensitive clinical practice. *Spirituality in Clinical Practice, 3*(4), 221.

Stone, B. M., & Parks, A. C. (2018). Cultivating subjective well-being through positive psychological interventions. In E. Diener, S. Oishi, & L. Tay (Eds.), *Handbook of well-being*. DEF Publishers (Noba Scholar). https://bit.ly/31EKhvE

Thomas, J., & Barbato, M. (2020). Positive religious coping and mental health among Christians and Muslims in response to the COVID-19 pandemic. *Religions, 11*(10), 498.

Walsh, R. (2011). Lifestyle and mental health. *American Psychologist, 66*(7), 579–592. https://doi.org/10.1037/a0021769

Waters, L., Algoe, S. B., Dutton, J., Emmons, R., Fredrickson, B. L., Heaphy, E., et al. (2022). Positive psychology in a pandemic: Buffering, bolstering, and building mental health. *The Journal of Positive Psychology, 17*(3), 303–323.

White, M. P., Alcock, I., Grellier, J., Wheeler, B. W., Hartig, T., Warber, S. L., et al. (2019). Spending at least 120 minutes a week in nature is associated with good health and wellbeing. *Scientific Reports, 9*(1), 1–11.

Williams, I. A., Richardson, T. A., Moore, D. D., Gambrel, L. E., & Keeling, M. L. (2010). Perspectives on selfcare. *Journal of Creativity in Mental Health, 5*, 321–338. https://doi.org/10.1080/15401383.2010.507700

Wise, E. H., & Reuman, L. (2019). Promoting competent and flourishing life-long practice for psychologists: A communitarian perspective. *Professional Psychology: Research and Practice, 50*(2), 129–135.

Wise, E. H., Hersh, M. A., & Gibson, C. L. (2012). Ethics, self-care and well-being for psychologists: Re-envisioning the stress-distress continuum. *Professional Psychology: Research and Practice, 43*, 487–494. https://doi.org/10.1037/a0029446

Wong, H. J., & White, K. M. (2021). A theory-based examination of self-care behaviours among psychologists. *Clinical Psychology & Psychotherapy, 28*(4), 950–968.

Wood, A. M., Linley, P. A., Maltby, J., Kashdan, T. B., & Hurling, R. (2011). Using personal and psychological strengths leads to increases in well-being over time: A longitudinal study and the development of the strengths use questionnaire. *Personality and Individual Differences, 50,* 15–19. https://doi.org/10.1016/j.paid.2010.08.004

Zahniser, E., Rupert, P. A., & Dorociak, K. E. (2017). Self-care in clinical psychology graduate training. *Training and Education in Professional Psychology, 11*(4), 283–289. https://doi.org/10.1037/tep0000172

Zhang, Z., & Chen, W. (2019). A systematic review of the relationship between physical activity and happiness. *Journal of Happiness Studies, 20,* 1305–1322. https://doi.org/10.1007/s10902-018-9976-0

Ziede, J. S., & Norcross, J. C. (2020). Personal therapy and self-care in the making of psychologists. *The Journal of Psychology, 154*(8), 585–618.

Zinn, B. B. (2022). *The flourishing trainee: Operationalizing self-care education in clinical psychology training programs* (Doctoral dissertation, Antioch University).

# Chapter 10
# Integration of Chapters: Applying a Systemic Lens to Clinical Supervision

In applying a systematic approach to clinical supervision that involves integrating the three different levels, it is envisaged that the supervisor and supervisee's practitioner's competence lens is strengthened. In this last chapter, I present an integration of the key themes that emerged from the various chapters. It is envisioned that at this point of departure, supervisees and supervisors will feel encouraged and supported to broaden their practitioner lens through reflection of the key themes highlighted.

## 10.1  Clinical Supervisor Competence Is Constantly Evolving

Falendar and Shafranske (2017) highlight that competency in clinical supervision is constantly evolving as the field continuously advances knowledge and professional practice. The traditional psychotherapy-based models that have dominated clinical supervision have largely promoted a biomedical, deficit approach to supporting supervisees. With the turn of the century, there is a need to shift the focus to systemic and integrated approaches, which include holistic, contextual and local indigenous perspectives that influence supervisee/trainee practice.

A systemic, ecological approach to clinical supervision advocated in this book presents how this can be facilitated at the different levels so that trainees can develop a greater state of cohesiveness in approaching consultation at different settings. In advocating for an ecological systemic approach, the author also acknowledges the expanding role Psychologists and health care practitioners have had to reconcile at practice settings such as primary health care facilities.

As highlighted in this book, integrating a systemic/ecological approach draws attention to systemic influences such as the need to integrate indigenous knowledge and skills in culturally complex and diverse countries such as South Africa. Clinical

K. V. Rawatlal, *Clinical Supervision in South Africa*, SpringerBriefs in Psychology, https://doi.org/10.1007/978-3-031-41929-4_10

supervision from an ecological perspective is seen to highlight the essential function of psychological training to, i.e. harmonise old and new Western, African and Eastern forms of psychological knowledge through exploring different world views. The assumption that while practitioners/supervisees recognise the need to intervene systemically, they often lack training or feel overwhelmed to intervene at the different levels. This publication has aimed to make it explicit as to the many ways this can be achieved and to some extent the need to account for the evolution that is needed in clinical supervision training and competence.

## 10.2   Level of the Core: *Humanness, the Personal Self in the Therapeutic Process*

At the *level of the core*, the focus is on acknowledging and strengthening the 'human-centredness' nature of the therapeutic alliance. Aponte (2022) states 'the personal self who is the therapist is an essential component of the therapeutic process because it is the human relationship with clients that is the medium through which the work of therapy is done' (p.136). Blow et al. (2007) also highlight that it is the therapist and not the therapy model per se that is more influential in the therapeutic process.

In the focus of this book which is based on the application of the ecological model to clinical supervision, there is a focus on the conscious and strategic use of trainee's use of their personal selves. The focus is on trainees being in touch with their own humanness to make strengthen connectivity (therapeutic alliance) with clients/patients. Through achieving consciousness of their own related personal struggles and vulnerabilities, (at the level of the core) practitioners are able to resonate and empathise with the distress and issues of the patient/client.

This level acknowledges both the personal humanity and social location in society of the therapist which includes the spiritual, philosophical, cultural, and socio-political dynamics of society which are all relevant to the therapeutic process which are all particularly relevant factors in navigating twenty-first-century realities that confront society.

The integrated approach advocated aims towards trainees adopting a sense of cohesiveness in therapists personal processes in relation to the psycho-social contexts in which they live and practice.

Sprenkle and associates (2009, p.4) stated

The qualities and capabilities of the person offering the treatment are more important than the treatment itself.

Carl Rogers (1961, p.44) also writes

It is the attitudes and feelings of the therapist, rather than his theoretical orientation, which is important.

## 10.2.1   Towards Self-Care and Well-Being

In focusing on the area of self-care and well-being, reference is made to research among South African university students that indicates they experience high levels of psychosocial vulnerability. Many students in SA are faced with several socioeconomic stressors resulting from the political history of the country that could impact their mental health, including widespread crime, gender-based violence, poverty, inequality, and housing and food insecurity (Beyene et al., 2019). The experience of trauma is seen to be associated with adverse mental health outcomes that include Post-traumatic stress disorder (PTSD), depression, anxiety and suicidal ideation. PTSD symptomatology (e.g. intrusive memories, persistent negative emotions, hypervigilance to threat) can impede a student's ability to engage with and complete academic tasks that require focused attention and cognitive flexibility and this has also been found to impact academic performance (Boyraz et al., 2016). This psychological sequela associated with trauma has been found to adversely affect psychological well-being. In South Africa, McGowan and Kagee (2013) assessed the prevalence of lifetime exposure to potentially traumatic events (PTEs among a sample of (N = 1337) of students at a large historically advantaged residential university. Approximately 90% of the sample reported exposure to one or more PTEs across their lifetime.

It is therefore important for supervisees to be cognisant of supervisees (student trainees) exposure to such events in communities and society at large. Clinical supervision also presents the space wherein there is an acknowledgement of supervisee's subjective vulnerabilities. It is therefore seen as important to encourage mental health professionals and supervisees to view themselves as being vulnerable to the personal and professional stressors of their career. This awareness of their own vulnerabilities is crucial so that supervisees can make a conscious effort to behave in ways that support overcoming or avoiding the cumulative effects of stress. The cumulative effects can lead to unprofessional conduct, unethical practices and malpractice complaints if not managed appropriately.

In relation to the above, in Chap. 4. Addressing the Core, I refer to the crucial role of self-awareness in supporting trainees in noticing and reflecting one's internal (individual) level and external experiences and monitoring one's own needs. This awareness of the self is highlighted as a conscious and continuous process that strengthens the therapeutic alliance through focusing on the role of the therapist. Self-awareness, located at the level of the core, allows trainees an identification with their own values and beliefs in motivating themselves to engage in behaviours that are fulfilling. Norcross et al. (2005) also encourage practitioners to revisit what initially led to choose a career in mental health in order to reawaken their sense of purpose and thus revitalise their spirit for the field of work. Supporting supervisees connecting and processing their personal struggles and vulnerabilities facilitates the ability to empathise with clients' and patients' struggles. This in turn, is also seen to play a role in strengthening resilience and the efficacy of clients/patients to overcome obstacles.

In including a dedicated chapter on *Wellbeing: Self-care in the supervisory space* authored by Tharina Guse, we hope to draw focus to the need to integrate self-care more proactively into clinical training programmes through clinical supervision. Self-care, promoted at the level of the core, through understanding self and the associated vulnerabilities/personality characteristics (highlighted in Chap. 4) allows supervises reflection and monitoring of their abilities to navigate client/patient presentations. This chapter should be read in tandem with Chap. 8, to allow supervisees to reflect on strategies/techniques to manage.

Robins et al. (2018) also highlight the need for self-care in training programmes making reference to the stress trainees experience and that may carry over into their transition to work. In Chap. 9 there is substantial support for the beneficial effects pf self-care practice in the reduction of negative outcomes such as burnout for mental health practitioners. Posluns and Gall (2020) highlight that among experienced mental health practitioners, self-care is identified as a key aspect of professional functioning. Dorociak et al. (2017) found that more experienced practitioners engage in more self-care behaviours and report less stress than practitioners who are early in their career.

The literature also identifies the area of self-care as being neglected. For example, many universities in Australia recommend creating and modelling a culture of self-care for trainees (Perry et al., 2017); unfortunately, self-care is often not formally taught or discussed within clinical training programmes. Roach and Young (2007) stress the importance of this aspect by indicating that students who are in clinical training programmes that promote self-care report greater benefits. The benefits of integrating the area are seen to have far-reaching positive outcomes in promoting positive mental health. The current literature suggests that a proactive stance toward self-care can help reduce negative outcomes experienced by mental health practitioners (Goncher et al., 2013) and improve the care of clients/patients (Schomaker & Richard, 2015). Both of these are regarded as ethical imperatives in the profession of health care.

## 10.3   Supervisee's Interactions with Interpersonal Systems of Influence

At this level, I highlight the role of the training, the supervisory experience, processes, and the role of the different psychotherapeutic approaches that supervisees are exposed to in supporting reflective ability and ultimately strengthening the therapeutic alliance. Attention is drawn to supervisees expanding their lens in provision of clinical supervision practice through making a shift away from the traditional, linear approaches to more circular and systemic approaches to supervision.

### 10.3.1 Shift Away from Medically Oriented Therapeutic Systems!

Implicit in applying an ecological systemic lens to clinical supervision is the assumption that a systemic approach yields more information for the Clinical supervisor to working with the supervisee and clients rather than working with individualised focused treatment models. Medically oriented therapeutic systems are seen to emphasise diagnostic and linear thinking that sometimes limit practitioner's ambit of interventions. A shift in focus from lineal to circular assumptions that is enabled through a systemic, ecological model emphasises a shift from lineal causality thinking to thinking which is relational and interactional in its assumptions. The merit of medically oriented therapeutic approaches however cannot be discounted, and practitioners (supervisees and supervisors) should be mindful that a complete shift away is not intended. The medically oriented therapeutic approaches are seen to support the work of Clinical and Counselling practitioners in points 1. and 2.

1. That is, that they support treatment and management of client/outpatient presentations (e.g. providing a diagnosis where required or facilitating access to medication – the work of Clinical Psychology) OR
2. They support identification of systems (mild/moderate/severe), behavioural modification and further referral to Psychiatry/Clinical Psychology – the work of Counselling Psychology)

### 10.3.2 Ethical Implications

Clinical supervision is internationally acknowledged to be the most important influence on psychologists' clinical practice (Orlinsky et al., 2005). It is regarded as the main means of instilling ethical knowledge, skills, and attitudes in a supervisee during the trainee process. Supervisors bear significant responsibility to their supervisees and clients; their highest responsibilities are to protect the client and the public; to ensure no unsuitable supervisees enter the profession; and to support and advance the development, competence, and ethical practice of their supervisees (Falender, 2000).

When supervisory training is offered, it is often facilitated through a psychotherapy-based model, which may not be systematic or include all the multiple components and dimensions of supervision (Falender, 2018; Falendar & Shafranske, 2010). Specifically, psychotherapy models may not systematically and directly address the supervisee's emotional reactivity and multicultural diversity dimensions. Integrating an ecological, systemic model supports supervisees consciously move through the different levels of development based on their interaction and reflection. This systematic approach to supervision supports trainees' identity and begins to monitor areas or levels for development to promote their growth.

Understanding supervisee socialisation and acculturation into ethical practice is essential. Supervisors need to be cognisant of how supervisees integrate their own personal ethics with professional ones.

Supervisors hold responsibility for both client care and for their supervises, and for understanding and integrating the worldviews and belief structures of the client(s), supervisees and themselves. The supervisor thus model's ethical behaviour, thus providing a hidden curriculum that is supported by multiculturally competent ethical practice. Supervisors should assess their own supervisor's competence, including understanding multicultural factors, modelling metacompetence, or considering what one does not know, and creating an environment in which communication and the supervisory and therapeutic relationships are facilitated. Acknowledging the limits of a supervisor's own competence and requisite the ethical steps to address those limits is seen as crucial (Falendar, 2000).

### 10.3.3  Ecological Oriented Clinical Supervisor Contrasted to Individually Oriented Supervisor

In integrating an ecological, systemic framework to clinical supervision, the author attempts to explore the question of 'What would the clinical supervisor do differently from an individually oriented supervisor? How would the clinical supervisor integrate the different layers?' The integration is facilitated through the clinical supervisor providing basic instruction in systemic concepts and their application at both the *individual* (supervisee's beliefs, motivation, personality, worldviews), the *interpersonal* (supervisee's relationship and interaction with supervisor, ability to engage in reflexivity, engagement with models/approaches to psychotherapeutic intervention) and the *institutional* (navigating the external reality/settings in which the supervisee's practice).

The need for such an integration is seen as apparent in navigating contemporary pressures and challenges that characterise practising in resource-constrained settings and institutions trainees find themselves in. Contemporary practice issues in the literature identify that increasingly secondary traumatic stress and vicarious trauma within the workforce are being linked with increase of feelings of burnout. Habeger et al. (2022) thus indicate the relevance of the socio-ecological model in providing a multilevel framework for addressing burnout and increasing resiliency among health care workers. As the ecological lens draws attention to several interdependent and interactional factors that include relationship with self, relationship with supervisor, the organisational and societal that influence clinician/supervisee well-being. This lens also provides a basis for understanding the aetiology of burnout and developing prevention and intervention practices (Habegar et al. 2022).

## 10.4   Supervisee's Interaction with the External Levels of Influence

In supporting supervisees navigate the challenges of working in resource contexts and settings, it is advocated through this publication that supervisees and supervisors need the awareness, skills and knowledge to intervene at *systemic levels* to address oppressive contextual factors that render clients and patients vulnerable and marginalised. A focus on systemic levels of influence enables practitioners to become aware of the significant role of the postcolonial and resilience-based/strengths-based frameworks in developing new approaches and frameworks that acknowledge the diversity of experiences and the integration of multiple ways of knowing.

### 10.4.1   Scientist-Practitioner Advocate Model

Consistent with calls for Psychologists to step outside of traditional scientist-practitioner roles this publication, through a focus on integrating a systematic lens, advocates for adopting a scientist-practitioner advocate training model. The addition of the advocacy component brings an explicit social justice focus on the roles of scientist and practitioner. It compels practitioners to study the impact of social issues and engage in systemic inquiry. Such a systemic focus engages the practitioner to work outside of the therapy room to reach out to oppressed or marginalised groups and seeks to empower clients and community groups to advocate for themselves.

At this level, I acknowledge the role of practitioner conscientisation through the training and supervisory relationship. Thus, contemporary, comprehensive graduate training must prepare students to intervene at both individual and systemic levels to effectively serve clients (Goodman et al., 2004; Vera & Speight, 2003). Thus, science becomes an act of advocacy in the best traditions of social action research (Lewin, 1948/1997). Fassinger and O'Brien (2000, pp. 263–264) argued for 'abandoning the illusion of scientific detachment and objectivity that is a legacy from the positivist model of science … all professional activities (research, teaching, training, consultation, supervision) are political acts that have social consequences'. This position is also supported in this publication through the promotion of a systemic lens to clinical supervision.

The self-awareness component of knowledge (discussed in Chap. 4) engages supervisees in continued self-examination of one's biases, emotional reaction stereotypes, and bases of privilege; as well as working to collaboratively share power with clients and give voice to those who have been silenced or suppressed (Goodman et al., 2004), rather than repeating the status quo of oppression. Reference is made to what Freire (2007) called 'conscientização', or 'critical consciousness', which includes the ability to 'perceive social, political, and economic contradictions, and to take action against the oppressive elements of reality' (p. 35), a habit of focusing on the strengths of individuals and communities, and desire to help clients develop tools that promote autonomy and self-determination. Building upon critical consciousness, through a systemic lens to clinical supervision, is seen as critical to developing supervisee's capacity to examine social context in thinking about clients' circumstances.

## 10.5   Conclusion

There is a growing awareness that the traditional domains of clinical practice are not sufficient to meet contemporary demands for graduates to be equipped not only to intervene and to study presenting problems at the level of individuals (or groups) but also at the level of systems. It is hoped that this publication, though 'turning the lens inwards' provides systemic support for preparing practitioners to meet the needs of clients/patients in a new century. Bronfenbrenner's (1979) ecological systemic model is seen as particularly helpful in conceptualising 'a systemic lens' to clinical supervision in different and diverse social contexts. Through the model's location of different levels of influence, it allows conceptualising competency, monitoring competency and skills development to strengthen the clinical supervision lens. Continuing efforts to refine and evaluate training through engaging practitioner's experiences of interventions provided through a systemic lens are necessary to support practice in resource-constrained settings and are deemed necessary to further inform practice in the twenty-first century.

## References

Aponte, H. J. (2022). The soul of therapy: The therapist's use of self in the therapeutic relationship. *Contemporary Family Therapy., 44*, 136–143.

Beyene, A. S., Chojenta, C., Roba, H.S., Melka A. S., & Loxton, D. (2019). Gender-based violence among female youths in educational institutions of Sub-Saharan Africa: a systematic review and meta-analysis. *Syst Rev, 8*(1), 59. https://doi.org/10.1186/s13643-019-0969-9. PMID: 30803436; PMCID: PMC6388495.

Boyraz, G., Granda, R., Baker, C. N., Tidwell, L. L., & Waits, J. B. (2016). Posttraumatic stress, effort regulation, and academic outcomes among college students: A longitudinal study. *Journal of Counseling Psychology, 63*(4), 475–486. https:// psycnet.apa.org/buy/2015-33093-001

Blow, A. J., Sprenkle, D. H., & Davis, S. D. (2007). Is who delivers the treatment more important than the treatment itself? The role of the therapist in common factors. *Journal of Marital and Family Therapy, 33*(3), 298–317. https://doi.org/10.1111/j.1752-0606.2007.00029.x

Bronfenbrenner, U. (1979). *The ecology of human development: Experiments by nature and design*. Harvard University Press.

Dorociak, K. E., Rupert, P. A., & Zahniser, E. (2017). Work life, well-being, and self-care across the professional lifespan of psychologists. *Professional Psychology: Research and Practice, 48*(6), 429–437. https://doi.org/10.1037/pro0000160

Falender, C. A. (2000). Education and Training in the 21st Century. *California Psychologist*, 18–20. Guest Editor of special edition on Education and Training in the 21st Century.

Falender, C. A. (2018). Clinical supervision: The missing ingredient. *American Psychologist*, 73(9), 1240–1250. https://doi.org/10.1037/amp0000385. PMID: 30525811.

Falendar, C. A., & Shafranske, E. P. (2010). Psychotherapy-based supervision models in an emerging competency-based era: A commentary. *Psychotherapy: Theory, Research, Practice, Training, 47*, 45–50. https://doi.org/10.1037/a0018873

Falender, C. A., & Shafranske, E. P. (2017). Competency-based clinical supervision: status. Opportunities, tensions, and the future. *Aust Psychol 52*, 86–93. https://doi.org/10.1111/ap.12265

Fassinger, R. E., & O'Brien, K. M. (2000). Career counseling with college women: A scientist-practitioner-advocate model of intervention. In D. Luzzo (Ed.), *Career counseling of college students: An empirical guide to strategies that work* (pp. 253–266). American Psychological Association. https://doi.org/10.1037/10362-014

Freire, P. (2007). *Pedagogy of the oppressed.* Continuum International.

Goodman, L. A., Liang, B., Helms, J. E., Latta, R. E., Sparks, E., & Weintraub, S. R. (2004). Training counseling psychologists as social justice agents: Feminist and multicultural principles in action. *The Counseling Psychologist, 32*, 793–837. https://doi.org/10.1177/0011000004268802

Lewin, K. (1997). *Resolving social conflicts and field theory in social science.* American Psychological Association. https://doi.org/10.1037/10269-000

Goncher, I. D., Sherman, M. F., Barnett, J. E., & Haskins, D. (2013). Programmatic perceptions of self-care emphasis and quality of life among graduate trainees in clinical psychology: The mediational role of selfcare utilization. *Training and Education in Professional Psychology, 7*(1), 53–60. https://doi.org/10.1037/a0031501

Habeger, A. D., Connell, T. D. J., Harris, R. L., & Jackson, C. (2022). Promoting burnout prevention through a socio-ecological lens. *Delaware Journal of Public Health, 8*(2), 70–75. https://doi.org/10.32481/djph.2022.05.008

McGowan, T. C., & Kagee, A. (2013). Exposure to traumatic events and symptoms of post-traumatic stress among South African university students. *South Africa Journal of Psychology, 43*(3), 327–339. https://doi.org/10.1177/0081246313493375

Norcross, J., Karpiak, C., & Santoro, S. (2005). Clinical psychologists across the years: The division of clinical psychology from 1960 to 2003. *Journal of Clinical Psychology, 61*(12), 1467–1483.

Orlinsky, D. E., Ronnestad, M. H., & the Collaborative Research Network of the Society for Psychotherapy Research. (2005). *How psychotherapists develop: A study of therapeutic work and professional growth.* American Psychological Association. https://doi.org/10.1037/11157-000

Perry, K. N., Donovan, M., Knight, R., & Shires, A. (2017). Addressing professional competency problems in clinical psychology trainees. *Australian Psychologist 52*, 121–129. https://doi.org/10.1111/ap.12268. [CrossRef] [Google Scholar]

Posluns, K., & Gall, T. L. (2020). Dear mental health practitioners, Take care of yourselves. A literature review on Self Care. *International Journal for the Advancement of Counselling, 42*, 1–20. https://doi.org/10.1007/s10447-019-09382-w

Roach, L. F., & Young, M. E. (2007). Do counselor education programs promote wellness in their students? *Counselor Education and Supervision, 47*(1), 29–45. https://doi.org/10.1002/j.1556-6978.2007.tb00036.x

Robins, T., Roberts, R., & Sarris, A. (2018). The role of student burnout in predicting future burnout: Exploring the transition from university to the workplace. *Higher Education Research and Development, 37*(1), 115–130.

Rogers, C. R. (1961). *On becoming a person: A therapist's view of psychotherapy.* Houghton Mifin.

Schomaker, S. A., & Ricard, R. J. (2015). Effect of a mindfulness-based intervention on counselor-client attunement. *Journal of Counseling & Development, 93*, 491–498. https://doi.org/10.1002/jcad.12047

Sprenkle, D. H., Davis, S. D., & Lebow, J. L. (2009). *Common factors in couple and family therapy: The overlooked foundation for effective practice*. Guilford Press.

Vera, E. M., & Speight, S. L. (2003). Multicultural competence, social justice, and counseling psychology: Expanding our roles. *The Counselling Psychologist, 31*, 253–272. https://doi.org/10.1177/0011000003031003

# Index